Get in Shape
FAST!

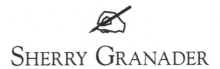

SHERRY GRANADER

Order this book online at www.trafford.com
or email orders@trafford.com

Most Trafford titles are also available at major online book retailers.

http://www.getshapefast.com

Printed in the United States of America.

ISBN: 978-1-4669-4924-9 (sc)
ISBN: 978-1-4669-4897-6 (e)

Trafford rev. 07/27/2012

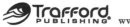 www.trafford.com

North America & international
toll-free: 1 888 232 4444 (USA & Canada)
phone: 250 383 6864 ♦ fax: 812 355 4082

Contents

Chapter 1

Eat Right . . . . Don't Diet!

Let's face it. Dieting is a dreaded endeavor, and according to most statistics, an expensive, wasted effort. Most diets fail most dieters. Most dieters fail most diets. Most diets imply starvation, not fulfillment. When hunger signals, the body is in need of nourishment and must not be ignored. To some people, hunger is a sign of feeling guilty rather than a time to fuel the body and enjoy some good food.

Throw out the diet, not the food! By learning to eat sensibly, developing ways to stay motivated, changing some lifestyle habits, and exercising, weight loss can be achieved fast. Those things may sound like lofty ideals prescribed by every fitness expert and health guru. Probably—yes, however, with knowledge of nutrition comes understanding. Strive to be wise consumers, informed cooks, nutrition experts, and fitness seekers. Don't throw out everything in the kitchen and start from scratch. That is unrealistic. Simply learn the principles of eating complete meals every 3-4 hours and learn to balance protein, fats and carbohydrates at those meals.

When most people go on a diet, the first thing they do is eliminate the carbohydrates. Potatoes, bread, and pasta become the enemy when actually, these foods in moderation give energy and when balanced with protein can lead to weight loss.

<u>Here is a breakdown of a complete meal</u>:

60% CARBOHDYRATES—this includes fruits, vegetables and whole grains mainly everything in the produce section or foods that are in their whole state.

20% PROTEIN—is needed to develop and maintain muscle tone.

20% FAT—each meal needs to include FAT—good fats like olive oil, macadamia nut oil, nuts and seeds like ground flaxseeds. Fat is necessary to keep our hair shiny and our skin youthful looking and our joints lubricated plus it is vital for the transfer of all the vitamins and minerals from our food into our cells, into our tissues for any health benefit.

This combination of protein, fats and carbohydrates in a complete mini-meal every 3-4 hours is the KEY to weight loss. There are so many FAD diets that people try that fail them. They may lose weight in the beginning but find the diet is impossible to stick with long term and so they go back to some of their old eating habits and gain the weight right back often gaining more weight than before they started the diet.

There are **3 FACTORS** for losing weight and keeping it off:

- **Eating Right** which this book will give you some easy tips to follow
- **Weight-bearing exercise**
- **Cardiovascular** training on the bike, treadmill or group exercise class.

Eating right starts with cooking right. Healthy food preparation must begin at home. Learn to cook tasty, low-calorie meals which are most of all, easy to prepare. For example, the fat in most recipes can be cut in half very easily. Use olive oil instead of butter, and find recipes without mayonnaise or sour cream. Sugar and salt can be deleted from most recipes and alternatives used instead like herbs, spices, flavored extracts and vinegars to make recipes delicious and appealing to the eyes.

If food doesn't look appetizing on the plate or table, it will not be eaten. Food should be a whole experience satisfying all the senses. Food presentation is very important. Make food look opulent by using the fine china or silverware. Dress up the table with a colorful tablecloth, fresh flowers and candles.

When it comes to eggs called for in recipes, use 2 egg whites for every whole egg called for in a dish. Egg whites are a major source of protein and can be made to look and taste the way eggs are expected to look and taste by using spices and flavorings. One YOLK contains 6 grams of fat so it is ok to add one whole egg to scrambled egg whites for example. Think FRESH, ORGANIC first when it comes to produce or fruits and vegetables, however, frozen works fine in a pinch or when certain produce is out of season.

Most people on traditional diets starve themselves to shed the pounds. Depriving the body of needed nutrients only leads to poor health. Dieters develop headaches, muscle pain, and weakness in the body. The energy level drops dramatically because of lack of nourishment. This makes it impossible to exercise when you have no energy. Dieting to lose weight without exercise or exercising to lose weight without dieting will not accomplish set goals. These 2 aspects must work together. The program must be balanced, like everything in life. Also, that balance is different for each individual.

When it comes to exercise, find a fitness facility that offers a variety of classes, qualified personal trainers and great equipment. Working out in a gym is fun, social, cheerful and motivating. You may want to check out local schools, colleges, YMCA's and churches for classes or special programs. CD's and DVD's are available for working out at home and of course, there is walking in your neighborhood.

The most important thing is to have fun and be consistent in whatever form of exercise you choose. The amount of exercise each person needs will vary, however, a program which features a 40-60 minute workout 3-4 days per week is a great beginning. It is important to do SOMETHING every day because you will find you feel better throughout the day and sleep better at night.

You will find exercise will do so much for you—reduce stress, increase strength and flexibility, give you energy, clear your head, reduce body fat and is the BEST way to slow down the aging process. Look for nationally certified Instructors and Personal Trainers and ask to speak to their clients for recommendations.

Chapter 2

Healthy Diet Mistakes When Your Healthy Diet Isn't So Healthy

Trying to eat healthier? Great. Just avoid these 9 common diet mistakes. The problem is, there is no quick fix when it comes to healthy eating. A healthy diet relies on a lifelong commitment to eating the right foods and eating the right way. You already knew that but many still go astray when trying to eat healthy. Here are a few of the "diet" mistakes people make and how to fix them before they derail your healthy eating plan.

1. One-Food Wonders

One diet promises that you can lose 10 pounds in a week by eating as much as you want—as long as what you're eating is cabbage soup. Or grapefruit. Or cookies. Bad idea. If you go on an extreme, short-term diet, you are setting yourself up to be very hungry and this can lead to bingeing.

By cutting out entire food groups, you're also prone to nutritional shortfalls and boredom. Eventually, you're going to crave the foods you're missing. Even when the diet works, it does not teach you how to maintain your weight loss. It's just a gimmick to restrict calories. Many of the "one-food" diets can also have some unpleasant side effects like dehydration, gas, depression and lack of energy.

Fix It: If a product or diet sounds too good to be true, it probably is. Weight loss should be a gradual process in which you lose no more than half a pound to 1 pound a week by eating a well-rounded diet.

2. Misguided Vegetarianism

More than 7 million people in the U.S follow a vegetarian diet and most of them do it with the best of intentions. Either they love animals too much to eat them, or they're opting for what they see as a healthier lifestyle. A healthy vegetarian diet has been linked to lower rates of obesity, diabetes and heart disease.

What many people don't realize is that vegetarian doesn't necessarily mean low-fat or low-calorie. If you're eating carbohydrate—or starch-rich foods, calorically, you might be eating more. In other words, if cheese, pasta, and smoothies are the foundations of your vegetarian diet, you can still gain weight and be unhealthy.

Fix it: Make vegetables the centerpiece of each meal. Add whole grains, fruit, and other healthy non-meat foods. Make sure you get enough protein from vegetable sources like beans, nuts, and tofu and essential amino acids from foods like brown rice.

3. Too Much of a Good Thing

A steady stream of research touts the benefits of one food or another. Chocolate, red wine, olive oil, avocados, and nuts have all had their day in the dietary sun. True, these foods have health benefits. But that doesn't mean more is better. For instance, chocolate, olive oil, avocados, and nuts are all high in calories. A friend of mine heard avocados are good because he had heart disease but he was eating three avocados a day. While they're nutrient-rich and good for you, he was eating at least 500 to 600 calories in avocados each day.

One tablespoon of olive oil has 120 calories. Red wine is alcohol, which in large quantities can raise your risk for heart problems and cancer.

Fix It: It's OK to add a healthy ingredient into your diet. But do it in moderation and as part of an overall healthy eating plan. That means a little olive oil, not a couple of glugs. Or a handful of nuts, not the whole bag. You get the idea.

What about so-called super foods, like the açai berry—an antioxidant-rich fruit from Central and South America—which supposedly have amazing health benefits? Take the hype with a grain of salt. The benefit of the food is only going to be as good as your entire diet. Different foods work synergistically for your entire health. The big picture is what counts.

4. Snubbing Carbs

On the flip side of the so-called super foods are foods that get demonized. If you purge your diet of them, you could pay a price, nutritionally. Carbohydrates are a prime example. You do want to cut down on white bread and white rice, because these and other refined grains are low in nutrients. The U.S. government's guidelines recommend that at least half of your grains are whole grains.

Fix it: Don't cut carbohydrates entirely from your diet. Carbs are the primary foods for energy. Whole-grain bread, oatmeal, and brown rice are high in fiber and rich in B vitamins like folic acid, which are nutritional essentials.

Fix it: If you want to lose weight, instead of going on a radical diet, make tiny changes in your life. Add more fresh fruits and vegetables to your meals. Eat a healthy breakfast every morning—a habit that research shows can help control your weight. Move more, too. Aim for 30-60 minutes of exercise into every day. Tiny little changes are the ones that will have the biggest results for your long-term health.

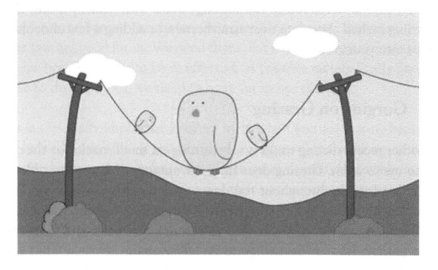

"Maybe it is time to change your eating habits."

Chapter 3

Setting Up
The Get In Shape FAST Program

The right combination of food is the key to success when beginning a low-fat eating and fitness program. Remember:

60% of each meal needs to be carbohydrates—whole grains, fresh fruits and vegetables—focusing on more vegetables than fruit. Keep your fruit intake to 2 servings per day. When it comes to vegetables, you can have as much as you want.

20% of each meal should include protein—lean meats like chicken, fish, tuna, salmon, egg whites or protein derived from egg whites or whey or in some cases, soy protein is acceptable

20% of each meal needs to be FAT—like olive oil, nuts, seeds, avocados are all good choices

For example, a boneless, skinless chicken breast = 6 grams of FAT
One Sweet Potato = 1 gram of FAT—add cinnamon
Baked asparagus drizzled with olive oil and seasoned with pepper = 2 grams of FAT

So you can see how easy it is to keep under the 10 grams of fat allotted for each meal. This combination of foods for each meal must be understood to enjoy a painless way to lose weight and feel great. High-protein diets alone FAIL because the balance of correct carbohydrates is not considered. You need carbohydrates for your brain to function. It is this balance of proper protein and carbohydrates with low-fat preparation and cooking that will take the weight off and keep it off. Add exercise and good health can be enjoyed.

If just a salad is eaten for lunch, hunger will attack in about 2 hours or less. At this point, the body is demanding something to fill a need and a fattening snack is what most people find to be the solution to the hunger. As long as the suggested balance of foods is eaten at each meal, hunger will not dominate. Healthy, low-fat snacks are allowed on this program as long as the total grams of fat does not go over 30 grams of FAT per day. Keeping within 10 grams of fat per meal will allow weight loss and maintenance for life.

Exercise including cardiovascular work and weight training will play an important role in your daily regimen. You want to do an exercise that will increase your heart rate for 30 minutes each day that will elevate your body temperature. This allows the body to burn up calories and burn off body fat. Exercise strengthens muscles and bones to help prevent osteoporosis.

Make an outline of a typical day of meals to note what time you eat breakfast, lunch, dinner, snacks, and what beverages are consumed. Do you eat alone or with other people and what types of foods are eaten at each meal? Make sure you include snacks as well as favorite restaurants frequented.

Many people skip breakfast or have only a piece of toast and coffee. Breakfast is a critical meal for many reasons. It sets the tone for the whole day. If high-energy foods are not eaten at breakfast, the body will demand something later in the day that usually comes in the form of a high-calorie, high-fat snack at mid-morning. If the day is started with sugar or just carbohydrates alone without any protein, it will set you up to crave more of the same all day.

A salad at lunch is not the answer to losing weight unless it has some good quality protein with it otherwise, you will be hungry again very soon after lunch and can lead to non-nutritious snacking. After not eating properly all day, it might make it easier to binge at dinner or be the prudent dieter and have only a piece of chicken or fish at supper. Either plan will fail.

This type of eating plan always fails a dieter. Instead of losing weight, health problems can develop including lack of energy, headaches, muscles pain, lethargy, high blood pressure or stress-related disorders. The frustration of being on a diet without success can lead to tension, depression and low self-esteem.

The right combination of foods at each meal is critical for the development of a healthy eating plan. Everyone is different and each plan must accommodate personal preferences, schedules and individual needs. You really do have to make time to eat! Think of your body as a computer. It only functions as well as what you enter into it. If you do not enter enough information or the wrong information, the computer will malfunction. Your body is the same! You must feed your body the right foods and enough food to keep it running at optimum levels.

Quick, low-fat meals that will stay with you for at least 3 hours are the key to preparation and success. You should look forward to your meals and not feel guilty when the hunger panes begin. Think of it as a time to fuel your body! You must eat—just the right way!

Chapter 4

The Get In Shape FAST Program

Eliminating the egg yolk from eggs is a good habit to get into—one egg yolk is fine to add to your egg whites. The fat in an egg is found in the yolk. Learning to cook with and eat just egg whites is an important part of the plan. Egg whites are a significant source of protein.

Remember the formula. For every whole egg, use 2 egg whites. Whenever a recipe calls for 3 eggs, use 6 egg whites. Egg separators can be purchased at most cooking stores to make separation easier and eliminate the risk of any egg yolk escaping into the food. When it comes to men, at least 6 egg whites should be consumed as part of their breakfast regimen that will enhance their efforts to support muscles and see results from their hard workouts.

There are many delicious and quick ways to prepare egg whites. One way to prepare egg whites quickly is using an egg poacher. Begin by filling the saucepan half-full with water and set on high heat. Spray the poacher cups with a little cooking spray and drop an egg into each cup. Season with a little sea salt and pepper to add great flavor and cover with the lid. Cook for about 3 minutes.

You can also add new red potatoes as long as you stick to the rule—eat the amount the size of your fist. Scrambling egg whites or making an omelet is another delicious way to prepare egg whites for breakfast. Fortunately, today egg whites are available in cartons in the egg section of most grocery stores. A great way to make egg whites is to heat a skillet on medium heat. Add some chopped onion, mushrooms, and tomatoes and cook for about 2 minutes or until the onions are transparent or caramelized. Add 1 cup of egg whites and scramble or you can make an omelet. Serve with Picante sauce for a low-fat, low-calorie, filling, tasty, colorful and nutritious meal.

Digestion of certain foods will increase the metabolic rate at different levels. For every 100 calories of carbohydrates consumed, a 10% metabolic increase can be expected. This is because **it takes more energy for the body to consume WHOLE foods than it does PROCESSED FOODS.**

Begin your day with WATER because after sleeping for 8 hours, your body is dehydrated and needs water to hydrate the body. Water is necessary for every process in the body so if you begin your day with coffee you are already at a deficit. Of course, still have a cup of coffee in the morning, however, it is important to limit your intake and avoid artificial sweeteners because they tend to increase hunger. To sweeten coffee, use Grade 'A'dark amber Maple Syrup which contains antioxidants and it takes very little to sweeten the coffee.

Make your egg white omelet or a quick meal for a breakfast is to make a Protein Smoothie with organic berries, ground flaxseeds, 1 cup soy milk and Nature's Plus SPIRUTEIN, ice and water. It is a good idea to take your vitamins in the morning to start your day right and make sure you are getting all the vitamins and minerals the body needs. The smoothie makes enough for a mid-morning snack so you can pour the rest into a thermos and take it with you to work and that takes care of breakfast and a mid-morning snack.

Another great snack is 8 ounces of Greek yogurt and add 1/3 cup of raw oats and 2 tablespoons of raisins or dried cranberries. Blend until well mixed. The oats help the body emulsify fat and the snack is very filling.

Since most people are in a hurry at lunch-time, it is important to find fast food restaurants that offer grilled chicken or shrimp salads or grilled chicken sandwiches that can be ordered with a low-fat salad dressing or with lettuce, tomato and mustard for the sandwich. Otherwise, make time for lunch and choose restaurants that you know you can have a healthy meal. Another option is to make your own lunch at home and bring with you in a cooler. Chicken salad, tuna salad made with mustard and relish is a good choice and you can add all sorts of vegetables like onions, cucumbers, celery, carrots, tomatoes and peppers. This will keep you full and you control what you are eating!

It is now 3-4 p.m. in the afternoon and time for another snack—my absolute favorite is a chilled, organic Pink Lady or Gala apple dipped in fresh ground almond butter. Almond butter is available at many whole food stores where they grind the nuts right there into small containers. The point here is to eat a snack. Make time. This is not an option.

The idea of eating dinner before six p.m. in the evening is unrealistic for most people because of people's hectic schedules. It is WHAT you eat after 6 p.m. that adds weight or body fat. Chicken, turkey, fish or another egg white meal with vegetables is always a good choice for dinner. If you are a meat eater or have one in your family, take a look at buffalo that is now available in most grocery stores meat sections.

Baked potatoes, sweet potatoes, salad, and or vegetables need to be added so you have a complete meal at dinner. Do not just have a baked potato and think this helps the weight loss cause. You must have a protein source, good carbohydrates like whole grains work well with a grilled chicken breast. Beans and rice work well for vegetarians with a tossed salad for a complete meal. For dessert, a piece of fruit or fresh strawberries make a great dessert topped with low-fat yogurt or check out some of the dessert recipes at the end of this book.

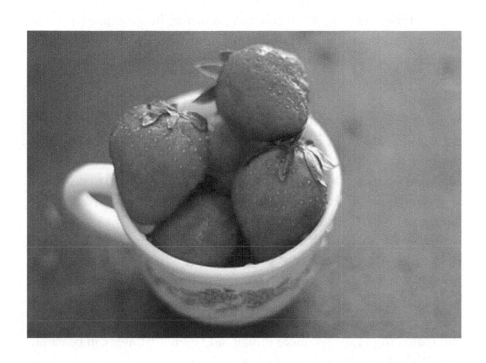

Chapter 5

Eat Right and Still Celebrate!

The best way to eat right not gain weight during holiday times is to eat as many meals as you would normally consume. Do NOT STARVE yourself all day and think gorging will be legal later at the big family dinner.

You will feel much better afterward if you don't skip any meals during the holiday season. A hearty meal at dinner can still be consumed if the prescribed intake of fat, protein and carbohydrates is adhered to according to schedule. You won't need to eat as much food to celebrate and your body will thank you later. Concentrate of the festivities with family and friends instead of focusing solely on food. Do not go to a holiday party hungry, otherwise, you may camp out at the buffet table.

It takes more energy to break down protein in the body before it is stored as fat, than it does any other nutrient. Carbohydrates are needed for energy and are either quickly burned or deposited as fat. If fat is eliminated from the diet, more protein and carbohydrates can be eaten with less risk of adding fat to the body.

If something fattening is consumed, it will see that the feeling of fullness is maintained longer. This occurs because the breakdown process of the protein and carbohydrates, plus fat, takes longer. If a low-fat meal is eaten with protein and carbohydrates, hunger will not hit for 2 or 3 more hours and fat will not be stored in the body,

Good sources of protein include egg whites, chicken, turkey, fish, buffalo, beans, legumes. Complex carbohydrates include sweet potatoes, potatoes, whole-grain pastas, rice, oatmeal, cream of rice, and vegetables. Simple carbohydrates include fruit, which elevates blood sugar level quickly releasing insulin. When fruit is eaten, it is better to eat the fruit with some protein like almond butter or peanut butter.

Eat protein and carbohydrates with good quality fats for a complete meal that will nourish the body. Do not skip meals! Find a routine that works for you and stick with it so it becomes a habit. When the holidays roll around again, you will be able to maintain your weight by sticking to your routine of eating complete meals every 3-4 hours combined with regular exercise.

Celebrations and holidays can sometimes lead to heartburn or acid reflux even with the best intentions of staying on your eat right program. It affects millions of Americans and many are treated with prescription reflux medications and although treatment is KEY to preventing further complications such as sleep problems, throat pain, irritability, hoarseness or chronic coughing, many would like to learn how to alleviate the burn without prescription drugs.

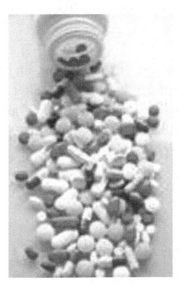

Here are some suggestions for the next time acid reflux sneaks up on you:

1. **SUGARLESS GUM**—Scientists in the UK found that chewing gum after eating a high-fat meal, reduced discomfort by 47%. This is because the repetitive chewing motion doubles the body's output of saliva that neutralizes excess stomach acid and flushes any spillover from the esophagus. Try STRIDE sugarless gum—it keeps its flavor longer so you can chew for 30 minutes after a meal.

2. **CANDIED GINGER**—this has been a well-known remedy for car-sickness but is also great for heartburn. Ginger contains active compounds like gingerol and ferulic acid that increases the production of bile and this stops the intensity of post-meal flare-ups. Keep candied ginger on hand or simply mince the candy and sprinkle it over some organic berries for a delicious dessert.

3. **GREEK YOGURT**—helps prevent reflux symptoms by giving your digestive tract plenty of probiotic (good) bacteria that are essential for proper digestion and absorption of food. For best results, choose organic yogurt because it contains 3 times more probiotics to fight acid reflux than conventional brands.

4. **ENZYMES**—help your body digest your food to prevent acid reflux from happening in the first place.

This is a good time to mention the endless health benefits of ENZYMES. They are especially helpful to have on hand after going to a celebration dinner where you may have eaten too much rich food for your body to digest. You may feel bloated and so full that you never want to eat again. Enzymes can help.

Here are some common symptoms of being enzyme deficient:

- Back weakness
- Fungus on toe nails or finger nails
- Constipation

- High blood pressure
- Insomnia
- Hearing problems
- Parasites
- Gum disorders like gingivitis
- Allergies
- Low energy
- Poor memory
- Fatigue
- Bloating, gas, diarrhea
- Digestive problems

If you are over the age of 40, you may be enzyme deficient which can prevent your body from absorbing the nutrients, vitamins and minerals from your food and experience good health. You are not getting old—you are running out of enzymes.

Enzymes are the catalyst that makes everything work together in your body. In other words, you cannot breathe, eat, drink, exercise or digest your food without enzymes. You cannot fight a cold or flu without enzymes. You have more than 3,000 active enzymes at work inside your body and they perform more than 100,000 functions to keep you healthy and alive.

Remember the energy you had as a child? This is because you had an abundance of metabolic enzymes to help create that 24-hour, non-stop energy! As we get older, we no longer have as many enzymes to digest our food. In fact, production of enzymes decreases about 13% with each passing decade. This is why certain foods that never bothered you before may bother you now—like spicy foods that tear up your stomach. It is also why a sports injury takes longer to heal and your thinking or memory may be foggy. Knees, back and joints ache constantly. I could go on and on but you get the picture.

Without critical enzymes, you may be creating a health problem without realizing it. You may think that poor circulation or a bad heart are to blame when in fact, it really is an enzyme deficiency. You may have heard about INFLAMMATION that has reached the headlines in many magazines and journals. TIME magazine calls inflammation "the secret killer" and it is true. Inflammation causes all sorts of problems, everything gets inflamed as we get older—our organs, tissues, joints, etc.

Enzymes can help:

- Reduce inflammation throughout the body
- Help lower cholesterol naturally
- Thin your blood just as well if not better than prescription drugs without side effects
- Absorb nutrients from your food and vitamin supplements so they work for you—not against you
- Improve joint pain

What ZAPS your enzyme bank account in the body?

- Poor eating habits
- Heating foods kills enzymes in the food itself
- Eating canned foods that destroy enzymes in the body and reduce the vitamin and mineral content in the food
- Frozen foods—blanching foods before they are frozen kills the enzymes
- Stress—causes your body to go into overdrive and forces the enzymes you do have work overtime
- Getting older decreases your enzyme production every decade so by the time you are 50 years of age, you may be enzyme deficient.
- Prescription drugs and over-the-counter medicines can damage or kill enzymes in the body

For more information about enzymes and their benefits, contact Transformation in Houston, Texas 800-777-1474. You will notice the difference in how you feel!

Chapter 6

How to Stay Thin Forever

Keeping weight down requires losing slowly and steadily, and most of all, being consistent with the Eat Right schedule and workout program. After making some simple changes in eating choices and adding consistent exercise, most of you will lose approximately 3-4 pounds the first week. Then, a weight loss of approximately 1 pound per week can be expected. It is important to some sort of exercise each day, whether it is weight training, taking a Yoga, Pilates or Aerobics class, or simply walking. Exercise is critical. Think about this formula:

Eating right + Exercise = Energy and Weight Loss.

Successful eaters do CHEAT—plan a cheat day! It means you can choose a day to eat whatever you want at every meal or all day and simply return to your regular healthy eating habits the very next day. Be warned! Cheating on a decadent meal, for example, will make the body rebel. No matter how wonderful the food tastes going down, once the body has adjusted to eating with the proper balance of good healthy food, the shock of those excess calories, fat and sugar will be difficult to tolerate.

If it is not a cheat day, and the need for something forbidden is felt, treat yourself to a low-fat version or instead of eating a fattening food, purchase a new workout outfit. Looking good and feeling good when you exercise makes it more fun! Learn to treat yourself without using food. Find a special place to alleviate stress. Seek surroundings that are peaceful and beautiful for you. Take time to be pampered.

There is so much pressure on women to look like the women who grace the fashion magazines and are in the endless array of infomercials and television shows. Have you asked yourself—how do they do it? How do they stay slim and fit? It takes more than scheduling workouts at the gym and gulping down a mug of coffee on the way to work. It will not sustain you for very long.

Here are some suggestions for staying slim and healthy at the same time:

1. **STICK TO A ROUTINE**—this means find foods that work for you and will keep you full without increasing your waist line. You have to take the guesswork out of eating your meals, especially breakfast and lunch. It might be egg whites scrambled with vegetables every morning and a grilled chicken salad for lunch—EVERYDAY! You might change the ingredients just a bit by making an omelet instead or substituting salmon for grilled chicken. Develop a routine that makes eating right a HABIT rather than a daily battle.

2. **EAT 'SOMETHING' BEFORE GOING OUT TO DINNER OR A PARTY**—going out to dinner or to a party is a part of life and if you eat well during the day, it will allow you a little room when ordering off the menu. Do not arrive at any restaurant starved otherwise you might devour the entire bread basket before the salad arrives. Order an appetizer for your entrée or ask if anyone at the table would like to split or share a meal or a couple of appetizers—that way you can taste some amazing dishes without really splurging.

3. **KNOW WHAT TO DO AT PARTIES**—all those delicious hors d'ouevres can pack on the pounds faster than you may think so make a point of holding a clutch purse in one hand and a glass of wine in another hand—that way you do not have any hands free to nibble.

4. **ALWAYS TAKE FOOD WITH YOU WHEN YOU TRAVEL**—Do not go anywhere without food. You can always find a piece of fruit, nuts or a protein bar so when the cart starts coming down the aisle with nothing but processed foods, it makes it easier to just order water with lemon or tomato juice.

5. **DO NOT ALLOW YOURSELF TO GET HUNGRY**—before you start feeling those pangs of hunger, take some time to eat ½ of a protein bar and take your time eating it. It takes a little while for your body to register that it is full and satisfied so do not rush it!

6. **EXERCISE**—no matter what, find time to exercise in your day. Wake up every morning and figure out when you can exercise by taking a Pilates class or doing Yoga or lifting weights or getting on the treadmill. MAKE EXERCISE A PRIORITY and NOT AN OPTION. Would you think of going through a day without brushing your teeth or taking a shower? Think about making the time to exercise and find something you enjoy doing and look forward to even if it is only 20 minutes of Yoga, for example.

7. **CONSISTENCY IS KEY**—do whatever it takes to stick with your plan. There are always going to be distractions or issues that arise so always have a Plan B.

8. **TREAT YOURSELF**—if you are going to CHEAT, indulge in foods that are totally worth it. If you really want dessert, the low-fat version doesn't always fit the bill or satisfy the craving. Instead have a small portion of the 'real' thing. You will find that you appreciate it more when you have it in moderation.

Chapter 7

Tips for Eating Right

EAT! You must eat to lose weight. When you don't eat, your body immediately goes into a defensive mode and thinks, "I better store this food as fat, because I will need energy later and I do not always know when I am going to get fed." That is your body talking! Eat from the earth! High volume, whole foods will keep you full and you will not be hungry.

Don't count calories—It's boring and who has the time. If you are on a 1,000 calorie a day diet and those calories were all consumed in the form of chocolate chip cookies, and you would feel terrible and lack nutrients. Again, eat from the earth and you will not have to worry about counting calories.

Set Goals—Do not expect to lose weight immediately. Pounds do not accumulate overnight, so do not expect to lose weight over night. Women who have gone through my Eat Right Program lose about 3 pounds the first week and then continue to lose about a pound per week if exercise is part of their schedule. It takes time to change eating habits, so take it one meal at a time! For example, if you are someone who skips breakfast all the time, let's start there! If soft drinks are your downfall, make an effort to cut down on their consumption. Personalize your program.

Be a wise consumer—Read labels carefully. Do not just read the front of the label. Fat and sodium content in foods can be particularly confusing. FDA has required strict labeling nowadays to guarantee food product label accuracy.

For example:

- Reduced calorie means that a product must have 1/3 fewer calories than a regular product.
- Low-fat means that a product must have 1/3 less fat than the full-fat version
- Be aware of serving size because a serving might be just a ½ cup and depending on the product, you might be consuming a lot more than a ½ cup.

Exercise! Exercise is a must. Find an activity you enjoy and not dread and do it! You will be amazed how well you feel, how well you sleep, how well you look, how much energy you have and how well your clothes fit. Your attitude will change and you will lose inches. It may not show up on the scale, especially if you are weight training because muscle weighs more but eventually you will lose inches all over your body. Your local gym or fitness center is a wonderful place to exercise, make friends, get personalized training and lose weight in the process.

Steam vegetables—it is a great way to keep the nutrients in the vegetables instead of boiling them in water where the nutrition is lost.

Serve your family the same meal as you would eat yourself—in other words, do not prepare them a high-fat meal and then you eat something else. The whole family will benefit from low-fat, healthy cooking and your children will learn a lifetime of healthy cooking habits.

Do not skip meals—take the time to eat. Eat mini-meals every 3-4 hours throughout the day. A Mini-meal consists of approximately 300-400 calories and always includes a protein source and fibrous carbohydrates.

Stay away from soft drinks! Regular soft drinks have enough sugar content for an entire day and contain a lot of caffeine. Diet soft drinks contain aspartame and other artificial sweeteners that can cause headaches and actually promote hunger. Why? Your brain registers that you received something sweet and your stomach says "where is it?" Your body is saying you told me I had something sweet and it is not here and many people report feeling hungry within an hour of consuming a diet soft drink.

Learn to <u>NOT</u> look at the menu at restaurants—this is an old trick of a bodybuilder friend of mine who makes of point of choosing restaurants where she can always get a grilled chicken breast or fish, a sweet potato and some grilled or steamed vegetables. If you look at the menu, it all looks so good, especially if there are pictures in the menu—it is too tempting to think to yourself—"I haven't had that in a long time" or you just plain can't resist ordering something decadent. She will look up at the waiter or waitress and ask "do you have chicken?" and of course, the wait person says "yes" and she will say "great—I will take that grilled" and do you have sweet potatoes? And typically they do—if not she will order the vegetables and a salad with the dressing on the side.

Chapter 8

Grocery Shopping List

Good eating habits begin with a trip to the grocery store. Have items on hand to make low-fat, healthy cooking easy and quick. This list will help the initial reorganization of your pantry and kitchen. If these items are staples in your home, it will make it easier to substitute healthier items in family favorite recipes. In other words,

IF YOU BUY EVERYTHING ON THIS LIST, YOU CAN MAKE EVERYTHING IN THIS BOOK!

Chicken breast—boneless and skinless
Turkey—rotisserie-roasted are good to have on hand
Fish, shrimp, crabmeat
Buffalo

Eggs
Egg White in the carton
Buttermilk
Soy milk
Fat-free and low-fat yogurt
Romano cheese
Parmesan cheese
Non-fat mozzarella
Non-fat sharp cheddar
Low-fat cream cheese
Brown rice
Low-sodium rice mixes

Couscous
Whole-grain pasta

Cream of rice
Oats
Oat flour
Rice flour
Whole-grain flour

Dijon mustard
Regular mustard
Hot pepper sauce
Mayonnaise made with Olive Oil
Picante sauce
Low sodium soy sauce
Low-sodium teriyaki sauce
Worchestershire sauce
Maple syrup
Molasses
Honey
Ketchup
Rice wine vinegar
Balsamic vinegar
Corn Starch
Baking powder and baking soda
Cooking spray
Lemons
Anchovy paste
Extra virgin olive oil
Italian herbs
Basil
Cayenne pepper
Powdered mustard

Thyme
Cilantro
Garlic
Oregano
Onion powder
Paprika
Poultry seasoning
Parsley
Fines herbs
Fresh dill
Cardamon
Rosemary
Vanilla extract
Simply potatoes (in refrigerated section near eggs)
Whole organic strawberries (frozen)
Frozen vegetables
Spreadable fruit
Raisins
Pizza crust
Bread Crumbs
Whole-grain bread
Baked Chips
Low-sodium chicken broth
Whole potatoes (red and sweet)
Italian tomatoes
Green onions
Celery
Bell peppers—red and green
Bananas
Apples (organic)

Chapter 9

Exercise, Weight Training and Cardiovascular

Instead of solely focusing on weight or measurements, focus on your total health. It is much more fun to focus on your total health, how you look and feel inside, how your clothes are fitting instead of going by the scale. When the scale doesn't indicate immediate results, it is too easy to become discouraged and abandon the program. The weight loss will come, steadily and gradually.

When we were young, our bodies burned calories and fat just by being alive. However, as we age, we burn fewer calories and store more body fat. The bottom line is that exercising at least 3-4 days per week is necessary to change lifestyles and become fit and lean.

Weight training will add more muscle mass to the body while creating a new shape. This additional muscle mass will add more weight to the scale weight, even though you will be leaner. The body proportions will change, and indicators given on typical weight charts will be inaccurate and misleading for your body type. To build endurance, start with a beginning weight—training program, using light pound weights with high repetition. (5-8 pounds dumbbells)

Cardiovascular exercise will help reduce body fat and the risk of heart disease, if the body temperature is raised for at least 30-40 minutes during each cardio session. Begin slowly, and gradually work up to optimum exercise level. This can be easily achieved by a difference in the music during the exercise period or a good way to shock your system rather easily is to do interval training. This is where you increase your speed on a treadmill for one minute and then return to your normal rate of speed. This is a great way to increase your metabolism and get results from your workout.

Below you will see a sample workout! The first workout for Monday is for Back and Hamstrings that focuses on 3 exercises for the back and 3 exercises for the hamstrings so we basically work the entire back of the body. This routine should be done once a week only for best results. On Tuesday, you have your choice of Yoga or Pilates class or possibly a Spin class. On Wednesday, we will work Chest and Biceps. Thursday is your choice of exercise. Friday is Shoulders and Triceps followed by Saturday that is an all-over leg workout. Sunday—REST!

Get In Shape FAST Weight Training Program

Monday: Back and Hamstrings

Back:

1. **Lat Pulldowns**—warm up with light weight and do 20 repetitions followed by 2 more sets of 15 repetitions with one more plate added to the weight stack.
2. **Rowing**—this can be done with BANDS or if your gym offers a rowing machine, you can do 3 sets of 15 repetitions.
3. **Seated row**—keep your knees slightly bent and keep your elbows close to your body when you bring the handles in.

Hamstrings:

1. **Seated leg curls**—make sure you adjust the seat properly so your back is pressed against the cushion and keep you feet flexed as you curl the weight in.
2. **Leg Press**—again, keep your back pressed against the cushion and do the repetition slow and controlled
3. **Standing Leg curls**—using a strap around your ankle, curl your foot up toward your glute muscles squeezing your hamstrings with each repetition.

Tuesday: Your choice of Exercise class

Wednesday: Chest and Biceps

Chest:

1. **Bench Press**—warm up with the bar only for 20 repetitions and gradually add weight to the bar for 2 more sets of 15 repetitions
2. **Cable Cross-Overs**—make sure you stand with your feet shoulder width apart and keep your elbows slightly bent.
3. **Flys**—these can be done on a machine designed for doing chest flys or you can use dumbbells

Thursday: Your choice of exercise class or treadmill

Friday: Shoulders and Triceps

Shoulders:

1. **Shoulder Press**—warm up with light weight and do 20 repetitions
2. **Pitcher Pours**—use light dumbbells and begin with the weights in front of you and take them out to your side as if you were pouring water out of the them using a slight twist on the way out
3. **Rear Deltoid**—You can use a Rear Deltoid Machine or dumbbells

Saturday: LEGS

1. **Leg press**—is a good machine to warm up with light weight and do 20 repetitions
2. **Leg Extensions**—work the quadriceps
3. **Hyperextensions**—focus on the glutes—check with a qualified Personal Trainer at your gym to show you these exercises properly. Form is KEY!

Sunday: REST! Rest is when you get results! Rest is when you give your muscles a chance to heal after you have worked the muscle hard and you will notice an increase in strength as you progress. Enjoy!

Chapter 10

Breakfast Recipes

Breakfast should always be eaten and enjoyed and can be one of your favorite meals. Eating breakfast will help keep your weight down and energy levels up. Make time for breakfast! By changing some old habits and experimenting with new recipes, you can start the day off right with any one of these breakfast entrees. Don't forget to take your vitamin and mineral supplements at breakfast time to maximize their benefits for the day.

CRUSTLESS QUICHE

This dish can be prepared ahead of time and eaten for breakfast or for any meal. In traditional quiche recipes, there is usually a lot of cream and fat found in the crust. By eliminating the crust, using egg whites and soy milk you can create a high-protein, low-fat version to be served for breakfast, lunch or dinner. You can serve a side salad with a Lemon-Vinaigrette for a delicious, filling meal any time of day!

1 package frozen spinach, chopped or one bag fresh spinach
½ cup green onions
1 tsp. Sicilian Herbs
1 cup of low-fat sharp cheddar cheese

In a blender: combine
1 cup of rice flour
6 egg whites
½ cup Soy Milk
1 cup of water
1 ½ tsp. Dijon Mustard
¼ cup low-fat Miracle Whip or mayonnaise

If using frozen spinach, remove foil wrapping and microwave for 5 minutes—drain. Combine with remainder of ingredients and pour into a quiche pan coated with cooking spray. BAKE at 400 degrees for 40 minutes. Remove and let stand for 5 minutes before slicing.

295 calories per serving
3 grams FAT
42 grams carbohydrates 12 grams of protein

Makes 6-8 servings

BANANA PANCAKES

6 egg whites
2 cups oat bran flour
1 cup of oats
2 bananas—ripe
11/2 cups of water
1 tsp. cinnamon
1 tsp. cardamom

In a large mixing bowl, mash bananas with the back of a large spoon. Add remaining ingredients and let stand for a few minutes. Coat a large skillet with cooking spray and turn on medium high heat. Pour about 1/3 cup of batter for each pancake. When the edges are firm and the batter is bubbling, turn each pancake and cook for another minute or two. Remove and serve with peanut butter spread on top for a high protein, filling breakfast.

210 calories for 2 pancakes
4 grams fat
12 grams protein
42 grams carbohydrates
Makes 12 pancakes

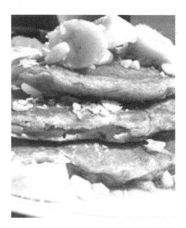

http://www.flickr.com/photos/santos/5785004/

GINGERBREAD WAFFLES

These waffles make a favorite treat for Sunday morning or for entertaining breakfast guests. The aroma is wonderful! It is gingerbread without a lot of fat and calories. Top with peaches, your favorite fruit or good old-fashioned Maple Syrup.

1 ¼ cup Whole Grain Flour
1 tsp. baking powder
1 tsp. baking soda
1 tsp. ground ginger
1 tsp. ground cinnamon
¼ cup Sugar in the Raw
6 egg whites
1 cup of buttermilk
½ cup molasses

Preheat Waffle Iron!

Combine first 6 ingredients and set aside in a large bowl. In another bowl, combine egg whites, buttermilk and molasses and mix well. Add to flour mixture and stir until well-blended. Bake in a preheated waffle iron coated with cooking spray for each waffle.

150 calories per waffle
2 grams of fat
32 grams carbohydrates
6 grams of protein

Makes 6 large waffles or 12 small waffles

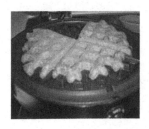

APPLE OATCAKES

To spice up regular oatcakes, I add chopped fresh apples to the batter—you can chop them quickly in a food processor. Top them with applesauce and serve them with some egg whites for a complete, lasting and nutritious breakfast.

6 egg whites
2 cups oat bran flour
1 cup of oats
1 ½ of cups water
Juice of half a lemon
2 tsp. cinnamon
2 tsp. apple pie spice pinch of nutmeg
3 apples—cored and chopped in food processor

In a large bowl, combine the first 6 ingredients. Chop the apples or use a food processor and add to the batter. Let stand for about 15 minutes. Coat a large skillet with cooking spray on medium high heat. Drop 1/3 cup of batter into skillet for each apple oatcake. Cook until the edges are firm and batter is bubbling in the center evenly. Turn and cook 2 minutes on the other side. Remove and serve with applesauce or fresh apple slices.

195 calories
1 gram fat
32 grams carbohydrates
6 grams protein

Makes 12 pancakes

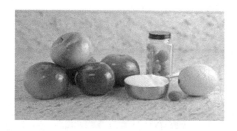

BREAKFAST BURRITOS

Choose whole-grain tortillas because they are high in fiber and low in fat. Wrap it up and take it with you for a delicious meal on the run.

4 whole-grain tortillas
8 egg whites
½ red pepper—chopped
2 Italian Red Roma Tomatoes—chopped
2 green onions—chopped
½ cup mushrooms—chopped
1 8oz. package of low-fat Sharp cheddar cheese—shredded
Picante Sauce
Olive oil

Add 2 tablespoons of extra virgin olive oil on medium heat. Cook red peppers, onions and mushrooms for about 2 minutes—add egg whites and scramble until cooked through. Add chopped tomatoes and cheese. Place tortillas on a cookie sheet coated with a little cooking spray and spoon egg white mixture down the middle of each tortilla. Fold over and pour picante sauce down the middle of each tortilla and bake at 350 degrees for 10 minutes.

If you are in a hurry, you may skip baking them in the oven and enjoy the egg whites wrapped in the tortilla for a quick, nutritious breakfast.

80 calories
2 grams fat
10 grams protein
28 grams carbohydrates

Makes 4 servings!

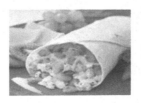

YOGURTS, OATS AND RAISINS

Keith Klein is a top Nutritionist who has helped many bodybuilders achieve their goals and win championships. This recipe tastes great, is easy to make and is an excellent snack.

8 ounces of low-fat yogurt or GREEK yogurt
1/3 cup of raw oats
2 tablespoons raisins

Mix all the ingredients together and let stand in the refrigerator for at least 30 minutes as it will set up and become firm. Otherwise, you can eat right away!

Greek yogurt contains less sugar and contains 3 times more Probiotics (good bacteria) than regular yogurt.

110 calories
2 grams fat
42 grams carbohydrates
3 grams protein

Makes ONE serving

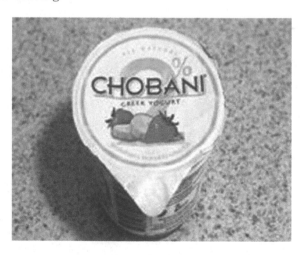

Egg White Omelet

I can make this omelet in a very short time for breakfast. Add a serving of oatmeal with cinnamon and raisins or a piece of whole grain toast with peanut butter or almond butter on it for an energizing, filling breakfast.

1 green onion—chopped
1 Roma Tomato—chopped
Handful of mushrooms—sliced
1 tsp. of chopped garlic
4 egg whites
Olive oil—one tablespoon
Sea salt and pepper to taste
Parmesan cheese
Picante sauce

In a medium skillet, add olive oil and set to medium heat. Add onions, mushrooms and tomatoes and season with sea salt and pepper—cook for about 2 minutes. Add garlic and stir quickly. Add egg whites and scramble or cook to form an omelet—top with Picante sauce or sprinkle with a little Parmesan cheese.

135 calories
2 grams fat
12 grams protein
18 grams carbohydrates

Makes one serving!

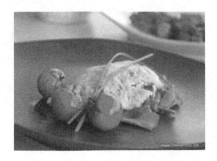

BREAKFAST POTATOES

My favorite way to make breakfast potatoes is bake a few potatoes in the oven the day before, let cool and refrigerate. I usually bake enough to last a week—they are delicious with breakfast or any meal.

1 potato—baked and cooled
Sea salt to taste
Pepper to taste
Olive oil

These make great seasoning options:
Sicilian Herbs
Onion powder
Pinch of fresh rosemary—chopped
Pinch of thyme

Heat skillet on medium heat and cut potato into even pieces. Toss with olive oil, sea salt, pepper to taste and your favorite herb choices in a bowl. Pour into skillet and cook about 2-3 minutes on each side. Serve immediately.

95 calories
1 gram fat
22 grams carbohydrates
1 gram of protein

Makes 2 servings

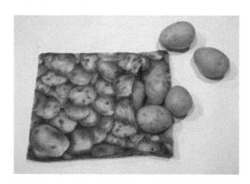

RASPBERRY FRENCH TOAST

Raspberries are one of my favorite fruits and this recipe is delicious to serve to family and friends for a special brunch or breakfast. Use raisin bread for an added flavor and top with fresh raspberries.

2 tablespoons Raspberry Spreadable Fruit
2 tablespoons low-fat Cream Cheese
8 slices of Raisin Bread
4 egg whites
¼ cup Vanilla Soy Milk
1 tsp. honey
½ tsp. vanilla extract
Cooking spray
Heat a skillet on medium heat.

Combine Spreadable fruit and cream cheese and blend well. Spread evenly over 4 slices of Raisin Bread. Top with remaining slices of Raisin Bread. In a bowl, combine egg whites, soy milk, honey and vanilla extract. Dip each sandwich into egg white mixture and place in a hot skillet coated with cooking spray. Cook sandwiches for 2-3 minutes on each side. Remove and serve with fresh raspberries and TURKEY APPLE SAUSAGE (recipe listed in my Main Dishes section of this book) for a real treat.

260 calories
4 grams fat
10 grams protein
32 grams carbohydrates

Makes 4 servings

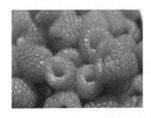

Chapter 11

Appetizers, Soups And Salads

There is no reason why entertaining at home must be done with high-fat, high-calorie foods. These recipes will help serve guests pleasing appetizers, soups and salads that are low in fat and calories without sacrificing taste or appearance.

STUFFED MUSHROOMS

These are one of my favorite appetizers, however, the usual stuffed mushrooms are high in fat. This delicious recipe reduces the fat in the stuffing significantly, so enjoy!

24 large fresh mushrooms
1 package frozen spinach, chopped
2 tablespoons extra virgin olive oil
1 clove garlic—minced
2 green onions—chopped
1 package of low-fat cream cheese
½ cup of whole-grain bread crumbs
1 tsp. ground dry mustard
Pinch of ground nutmeg
Sea salt and pepper to taste
Parmesan cheese

PREHEAT OVEN TO 375 degrees

Clean all the mushrooms by wiping each of them with a paper towel. If you wash them, they absorb water very quickly and become soggy and tasteless. Remove the stems and chop them! Microwave spinach for 5 minutes and drain. Coat a baking dish with cooking spray and place mushrooms inside the dish.

In a medium skillet on medium heat, add olive oil and cook onions and garlic. Add mushroom stems and spinach and cook until heated through. Remove from heat and let cool. Combine mushroom mixture with cream cheese, mustard, nutmeg, sea salt and pepper to taste. Spoon mixture into each mushroom cap and sprinkle with Parmesan cheese. Bake mushrooms at 375 degrees for 15 minutes!

EGG WHITE CREPE CUPS

These crepe cups make a fun and filling way to present egg whites to your family and friends. They will never know how low-fat and healthy they are so go ahead and serve them for satisfying brunch.

6 Ready-made crepes—look for these in the produce section next to strawberries
8 egg whites
2 green onions—chopped
½ cup of low-fat shredded Sharp Cheddar cheese
2 Roma Tomatoes—chopped
1 tsp. onion powder
Sea salt and pepper to taste
Cooking spray
Paprika

PREHEAT OVEN TO 350 degrees

Spray a muffin pan with cooking spray and carefully place one crepe inside each cup—there will be excess at the top of each muffin cup. Evenly disburse chopped onions, cheddar cheese and chopped tomatoes in each cup. Whip egg whites with onion powder, sea salt and pepper and pour seasoned egg whites into each cup. Sprinkle with paprika and bake at 350 degrees for 35-40 minutes until golden.

80 calories per crepe cup
1 gram of fat
10 grams of carbohydrates
18 grams protein

Makes 6 servings

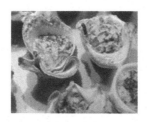

BAKED NEW RED POTATOES

Baking new red potatoes at a high temperature will yield delicious appetizers that are crispy on the outside and moist and meaty on the inside. Serve an arrangement of low-fat condiments for potato toppings and allow 2 potatoes per person.

One bag of New Red Potatoes
Sea salt and pepper to taste
Extra virgin olive oil

TOPPINGS:

Low-fat shredded Sharp Cheddar cheese
Picante Sauce
Green Onions—chopped
Low-fat Sour Cream
Chopped parsley
Fresh lemon—squeezing lemon over a potato is tangy and delicious

PREHEAT OVEN to 400 degrees

Wash potatoes, pat dry and place in large bowl. Drizzle olive oil over potatoes and season with sea salt and pepper. Place on a cookie sheet and bake for one hour. When potatoes are done, serve as an appetizer or a side dish to any meal.

95 calories per medium potato
1 gram fat
22 grams carbohydrates
2 grams protein

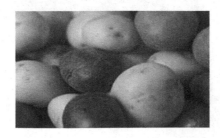

LOW-FAT FRESH VEGETABLE DIP

This dip is wonderful served with BAKED chips of any kind. This is definitely an indulgence and it can be prepared a day ahead of a party for convenience.

1 10-ounce package of frozen chopped spinach
1 cup of low-fat plain GREEK yogurt
2 tablespoons of fresh lemon juice
½ cup minced parsley
2 green onions—chopped
¼ cup low-fat Miracle Whip
1 tsp. fines herbs
1 tsp. minced fresh dill
Sea salt and pepper to taste
Paprika

Thaw frozen spinach or microwave for 5 minutes, drain and let cool. Squeeze the spinach dry and transfer into a bowl. Add remaining ingredients, except paprika. Mix well and refrigerate. Sprinkle paprika over the top in your favorite serving bowl.

60 calories per one cup
2 grams fat
22 grams carbohydrates
9 grams protein

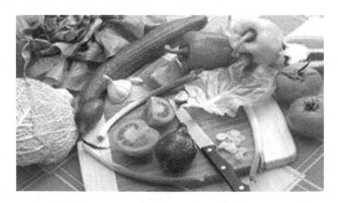

PEANUT BUTTER VINAIGRETTE

This is by far one of my favorite salad dressings to make—it is so easy to prepare and does not need refrigeration. Make enough to last a couple of days and store in an air-tight container.

In a bowl, add:

3 tablespoons of peanut butter—preferably organic or fresh ground
3 tablespoons Rice Wine Vinegar
1 tablespoon of honey
1 tablespoon of low-sodium Soy sauce
1 tablespoon Toasted Sesame Oil
1 tsp. ground ginger
Pinch of red pepper

Whisk together until all ingredients are blended smooth. Toss with your favorite greens—Romaine works well with this dressing. Add toasted almonds, dried cranberries, tomatoes, onions, pistachio nuts, etc. for a delicious salad any time of day.

BALSAMIC VINAIGRETTE

Once you get used to making your own salad dressings at home, you will not want to use store bought salad dressing any more. Here is another favorite!

In a bowl, add:
¼ cup balsamic vinegar
2 tablespoons Dijon Mustard
1 shallot—chopped
½ cup extra virgin olive oil
Sea salt and pepper to taste

Toss with Bibb lettuce, tomatoes, cucumbers, green onions and your favorite salad ingredients for a great-tasting salad.

PARTY TURKEY MEATBALLS

These make a great appetizer and are low in fat by using ground turkey breast. Take advantage of store-bought 'Simply Potatoes' in this recipe for added convenience. The meatballs can be made ahead and frozen without the sauce.

2 pounds ground turkey breast
½ cup Simply Potatoes—shredded
2 egg whites
1 bottle Chili Sauce
4 tablespoons Grape spreadable fruit
1 tablespoon Worcestershire Sauce
Sea salt and pepper to taste

Combine first 4 ingredients in a bowl—Season with salt and pepper. Form into meat balls and set aside. In a large skillet, combine chili sauce, Worcestershire sauce and grape Spreadable Fruit. Add meatballs and cover. Turn heat to low and cook for 30 minutes. Stir occasionally. When ready to serve as an appetizer, transfer to a chafing dish to keep warm.

35 calories per meatball
1 gram fat
6 grams protein
10 grams carbohydrates

Makes about 50 meatballs

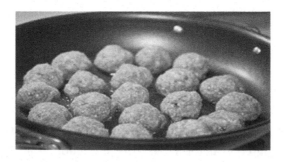

LOW-FAT SPINACH BALLS

Party guests love these appetizers and no one will realize how low-fat they are—you can make them ahead of time and freeze.

12 egg whites
2 packages frozen chopped spinach
2 cups herb stuffing mix
3 green onions—chopped
½ cup Parmesan cheese—shredded
1 tsp. Poultry seasoning
Sea salt and pepper to taste

PREHEAT OVEN TO 350 degrees

Beat egg whites in a large bowl and add remaining ingredients—form into 1 ½ inch size balls and place on a cookie sheet. BAKE for 20 minutes at 350 degrees.

35 calories per meatball
1 gram fat
11 grams carbohydrates
2 grams protein

Makes about 6 dozen

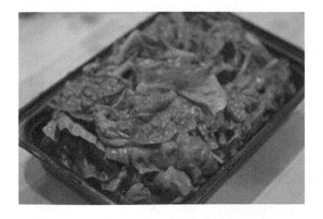

CRAB CAKES WITH RED PEPPER SAUCE

I had to develop a low-fat version of this classic appetizer. The sauce is so easy to make and your family and friends will think you slaved in the kitchen for hours.

1 pound of lump crab meat
1 shallot—chopped finely
1 tablespoon of whole-grain flour or rice flour
4 egg whites—lightly beaten
2 green onions—finely chopped
1 cup Italian Rice Bread Crumbs
1 tablespoon chopped fresh parsley
1 tablespoon chopped fresh dill
Cooking spray
Extra virgin olive oil
Sea salt and pepper to taste

In a large skillet, cook shallots for a minute or two in extra virgin olive oil on medium heat. Remove from heat and set aside. Combine crab meat with remaining ingredients including shallots. Heat skillet again and form patties with the crab meat mixture and cook about 3-5 minutes on each side. Serve immediately with Red Pepper Sauce—see below.

RED PEPPER SAUCE

This sauce is so easy to make that I always keep the ingredients on hand to make any time—it goes well with crab cakes, seafood and even chicken.

1 jar of Roasted Red peppers—drain
1 jar of Picante Sauce

Pour both jars into a food processor—transfer to a sauce pan and heat through.

To plate: Pour a ladle full of sauce on plate and move plate in a circular motion to cover the entire plate. Place 2 crab cakes in the center of each plate. Garnish with fresh parsley or fresh lemon slices.

COUSCOUS CHICKEN SOUP

Couscous is Moroccan pasta that can be found in the rice or pasta section of most grocery stores. It makes a great side dish or works well here added to soup.

1 large container of low-sodium chicken broth in carton
2 bay leaves
2 green onions—chopped
1 ½ tsp. of ground cumin
½ cup couscous
Juice of one lemon
Pulled cooked chicken breast—option

Simmer first 5 ingredients together in a large stock pot over medium heat for 10 minutes. Add couscous, lemon juice and cooked chicken and cook for an additional 5-10 minutes and you are ready to serve.

180 calories without the chicken
2 grams fat
28 grams carbohydrates
4 grams protein

Makes 2-4 servings

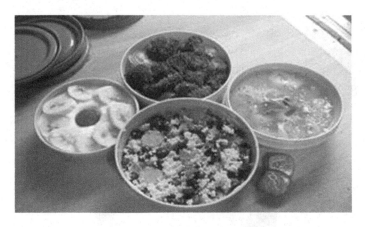

POTATO BROCCOLI CHOWDER

Since my childhood days in Michigan, Potato-Broccoli Chowder has always been one of my favorite soups. This is a low-fat version of the Midwestern classic using soy milk instead of cream.

2 packages of frozen chopped broccoli or 2 large heads of fresh broccoli—chopped
4 potatoes—baked and cut into small squares
3 green onions—chopped
1 clove garlic—minced
Extra virgin olive oil
4 quarts low-sodium chicken broth
½ cup of plain soy milk
Sea salt and pepper to taste

Cook broccoli until tender. Drain. In large pot on medium heat, add 2 tablespoons olive oil and cook green onions for about 2 minutes—add garlic and cook another minute. Add potatoes and cook for about 5 minutes, then add broccoli, chicken broth and soy milk. Season with Sea salt and pepper. Bring to a boil and reduce heat and simmer until potatoes are tender.

225 calories per cup
3 grams of fat
42 grams carbohydrates
12 grams protein

Serves 8

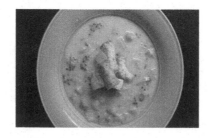

CHILLED CUCUMBER SOUP

Substituting low-fat yogurt for heavy cream in this recipe will cut the fat content significantly without cutting flavor and is a good tip for other recipes calling for heavy cream. This recipe is good to make ahead of time so you can enjoy it with a quick meal.

1 English cucumber—chopped
1 yellow onion—chopped
1 chicken bouillon cube
1 ½ cups low-fat yogurt—plain
1 tablespoon minced chives
Sea salt and pepper to taste
Fresh dill for garnish

Combine cucumber and onion in a medium sauce pan—add water to just cover vegetables and stir in bouillon cube—simmer until cucumber and onions are tender. Let cool, cover, and refrigerate. When ready to serve, blend in yogurt and chives and pour into serving bowls. Garnish with fresh dill or reserve some fresh cucumber to slice for the top of the soup.

80 calories per bowl
1 gram fat
12 grams carbohydrates
2 grams protein

Makes 4 servings

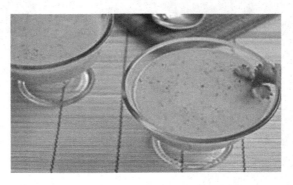

HEALTHY GAZPACHO SOUP

This soup is a summertime favorite because it is served chilled and is so good for you. Try this low-fat version for a spicy treat anytime of day.

4 ripe tomatoes—peeled and diced
1 cucumber—peeled and diced
1 green pepper—chopped
1 medium onion—finely chopped
1 clove garlic—chopped
1 cup low-sodium tomato juice or non-alcoholic Bloody Mary Mix for a spicy version
½ cup low-fat Italian salad dressing

Mix together all ingredients and chill for several hours before serving. Store in an air-tight container.

54 calories per cup
1 gram fat
12 grams carbohydrates
2 grams protein

Makes 4 servings

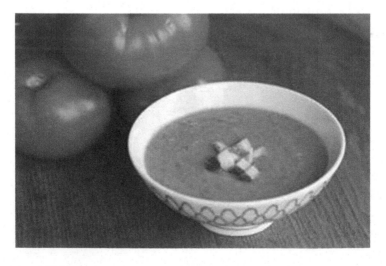

CHICKEN AND TORTELLINI SOUP

This is a great way to enjoy Italian food without a lot of calories and fat. It is great to make on a cold, winter day.

2 large cartons of chicken broth
1 package of tortellini stuffed with chicken
4 chicken breasts—cooked and cut into squares
½ pound sliced mushrooms
1 red bell pepper—chopped
1 cup brown rice—cooked
2 tsp. tarragon leaves—chopped

In a large pot, bring broth to a boil and cook tortellini and brown rice in broth. Add remaining ingredients and heat through until peppers are tender.

Ladle into bowls and sprinkle with Parmesan Cheese.
200 calories per bowl
4 grams fat
21 grams carbohydrates
19 grams protein

Makes 8 servings

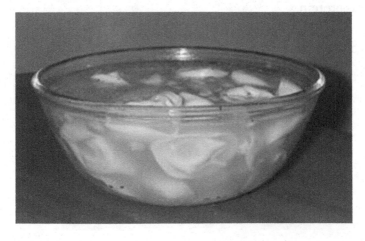

TURKEY RICE SOUP

Left-over turkey from Thanksgiving or any time you roast a turkey is great in this soup. Try it any time of year for a low-fat, healthy start to any meal or by itself.

2 large cartons of low-sodium chicken broth
1 cup of wild rice
2 cups turkey meat—cooked
3 stalks celery—chopped
4 green onions—chopped
1 can of low-sodium stewed tomatoes (14 ½ ounces)
1 tablespoon of ground sage
1 tablespoon of marjoram leaves
4 cloves garlic—chopped
2 bay leaves
Sea salt and pepper to taste

Combine all the ingredients in a large stock-pot and bring to a boil. Reduce heat and simmer until rice is tender.

245 calories per bowl
5 grams fat
24 grams carbohydrates
26 grams protein

Makes 8 servings

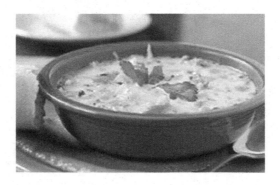

HONEY-MUSTARD SALAD DRESSING

Even though there are so many commercially made salad dressings on the market today, it is always good to be able to make your own from scratch with minimal effort. This dressing is great to toss with fresh spinach leaves and mushrooms. Garnish with low-fat shredded mozzarella cheese and chopped egg for a real treat.

1 large carton of low-fat plain yogurt
½ cup mustard
3 tablespoons honey
¼ cup Red Wine Vinegar
Dash of paprika
Sea salt and pepper to taste

12 calories per tablespoon
0.2 grams fat
24 grams carbohydrates
9 grams protein

Makes enough dressing for 4-6 large Spinach salads

LOW-FAT CAESAR DRESSING

It is hard to believe that a Caesar Salad could be low in fat and still taste wonderful. Try this version for yourself or family and friends for a great start or finish to any meal.

2 large heads of Romaine lettuce
1 cup sliced fresh mushrooms
¼ cup water
2 tablespoons grated Parmesan Regiano
2 tablespoons Red Wine Vinegar
1 ½ tsp. Anchovy paste
¼ cup olive oil
2 cloves garlic—chopped
Sea salt and pepper to taste

Wash lettuce and set aside. In a bowl, whisk together water, Parmesan, vinegar, anchovy paste, olive oil and garlic—Season with sea salt and pepper. Toss with Romaine lettuce and mushrooms.

37 calories per ½ cup serving
1.5 grams fat
8 grams carbohydrates
3 grams protein

Makes 4 servings

LOW-CALORIE COLESLAW

Cabbage, broccoli and cauliflower are cruciferous vegetables that are high in fiber and should be eaten as often as possible. This coleslaw dressing can be used with all three for a variation.

1 large cabbage or 1 bag of shredded cabbage
2 green onions—finely chopped
Juice of one lemon
¾ cup low-fat Miracle Whip
1 tablespoon Caraway seeds
Paprika
Sea salt and pepper to taste

Shred cabbage in food processor and place in bowl. Combine onion, lemon juice, Miracle Whip, caraway seeds, sea salt and pepper to taste. Chill—toss with cabbage just before serving. Sprinkle with paprika.

30 calories per ½ cup
1 gram fat
11 grams carbohydrates
1 gram of protein

Makes 6 servings

Chapter 12

Healthy Main Dishes

Eating 3 carrot sticks and a plain, boneless, skinless chicken breast is not my idea of a healthy dinner. It is starvation. Low-fat cooking can be convenient and filling without packing on the pounds. There are easy ways to substitute or eliminate high fats from most recipes if the ingredients are available to you in your kitchen for quick preparation.

Main dishes should taste wonderful, be easy to prepare and low in fat. Once low-fat substitution is understood, try re-writing your family favorite recipes! It is actually fun to do and good for you.

Nutrient-dense meals should become a priority in your life and your family's life to enjoy long-term health and wellness. The key to increasing your metabolism is to have foods or meals prepared and ready to go so you can eat every 3-4 hours or pack in a cooler to take with you to work.

Here are some recipes that you can make ahead of time and store in the freezer or refrigerator for a healthy meal any time of day!

CASHEW CHICKEN SALAD

This is a great recipe to make on a regular basis and keep in the fridge for a quick meal any time of day.

SALAD DRESSING:

1 tablespoon Cashew Nut butter
4 tablespoons Rice Wine vinegar
Juice of one lime
1 tsp. ground ginger
1 tablespoon minced garlic
1 tsp. lime zest
1 tablespoon toasted sesame oil

Whisk together ingredients until well-blended and set aside.

FOR THE CHICKEN SALAD:

2 cups cooked chicken—chopped
2 cups shredded Napa cabbage
2 green onions—chopped
1 cup diced carrots
1 cup diced celery
½ red bell pepper—chopped
1 fresh orange—cut into chunks
Fresh cashew nuts
Grape Size tomatoes

Combine chicken first 7 ingredients. Sprinkle cashew nuts on top of each serving of chicken salad along with grape size tomatoes. Store this salad in an air tight container in the fridge—if you add the cashew nuts to the chicken salad, they will become soft so I like to sprinkle them on top for added crunch!

PISTACHIO-BASIL PESTO CHICKEN

This is a great variation of home-made pesto using pistachio nuts for added flavor instead of the usual pine nuts and is wonderful on grilled chicken. It stores well in the freezer too.

1 cup shelled pistachio nuts
4 ounces of pine nuts
1 cup of fresh basil
2 garlic cloves
¾ cup extra virgin olive oil
Sea salt and pepper to taste

Toast the pine nuts and pistachio nuts in the oven at 350 for about 5-6 minutes on a rimmed cookie sheet. Let cool!!

In a food processor, combine all ingredients and season with salt and pepper.

You can use ice cube trays to freeze individual portions of pesto for a quick meal anytime. Spread on chicken or fish for a tasty entrée.

TOMATO-BASIL SAUCE

Make this sauce in large quantities to have on hand for making low-fat pasta dishes, chicken or fish and you can use it as a pizza sauce too—just add 2 tablespoons of tomato paste for a delicious pizza. This is the sauce for my Turkey-Spinach Lasagna on the next page. Enjoy!

2 large cartons of POMI tomato sauce with tomato chunks
4 cloves of garlic—chopped
4 tsp. ground oregano
4 tsp. Italian herbs
4 tsp. of ground basil or if fresh basil is available—chop 1 large bunch
1 cup Red wine—Cabernet Sauvignon works well

Pour ingredients in a large stock pot and bring to a boil. Reduce heat and simmer until ready to use for Turkey-Spinach Lasagna recipe or for your favorite Italian meal.

45 calories per cup
0 fat
10 grams carbohydrates

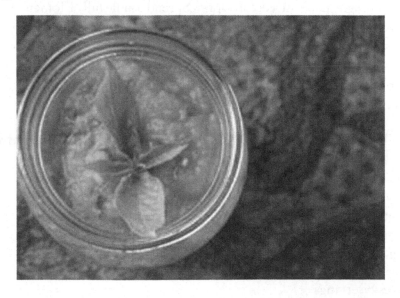

TURKEY-SPINACH LASAGNA

You can substitute buffalo for the turkey for a more filling variation.

2 pounds ground turkey breast, cooked
2 packages of frozen chopped spinach or 2 bags of fresh spinach
4 cloves garlic—minced
1 onion—chopped
2 tablespoons Extra Virgin Olive Oil
3 egg whites
½ cup Parmesan cheese
Sherry's Tomato Basil Sauce
1 package of no-bake lasagna noodles made from RICE
1 large package of low-fat mozzarella shredded
Cooking Spray

In a large skillet, cook ground turkey in a little olive oil and pour into large bowl. In same skillet, add a little more olive oil and cook onions until translucent and add garlic and cook for one minute. Add to turkey. Cook frozen chopped spinach and drain well. Add to turkey mixture. Add egg whites and Parmesan cheese.

Coat a lasagna pan with cooking spray. Spread a ladle full of Tomato-Basil Sauce on bottom of pan. Place one layer of lasagna noodles on bottom and spoon turkey mixture over noodles and sprinkle with Mozzarella cheese. REPEAT with noodles and turkey mixture. Finish with one layer of noodles and spread Tomato-Basil sauce over top. Sprinkle with Mozzarella and little more Parmesan on top.

BAKE for 45 minutes at 375 degrees. REMOVE from oven and let stand for 10 minutes before slicing.

450 calories per serving
6 grams of fat
45 grams carbohydrates
18 grams protein

Makes 8 servings

MARGHERITA PIZZA

This low-fat version of a favorite, Italian Pizza was created in honor of Italy's nineteenth century Queen Margherita. I add sun-dried tomatoes and use a Sicilian Blend of herbs available at most gourmet cooking stores.

1 THIN pizza crust—BOBOLI works the best!
Cooking spray
1 jar of PESTO or use the PESTO recipe in this book
8 ounces of low-fat mozzarella shredded
2 Roma tomatoes—sliced
½ cup sliced Sun-Dried Tomatoes
2 tablespoons of ground oregano or use a SICILIAN HERB BLEND
Chopped FRESH basil
¼ cup Parmesan cheese

PREHEAT OVEN TO 400 degrees

Spray a PIZZA pan with cooking spray and lay crust on top of pan. Spread evenly with pesto. Add sliced tomatoes and sun-dried tomatoes. Sprinkle with oregano herbs or Sicilian herbs and cheeses. BAKE at 400 degrees for 17 minutes!

SLICE and enjoy!

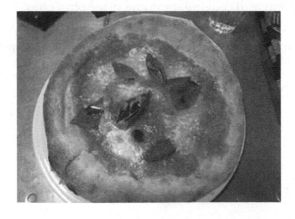

VEGETARIAN PIZZA

If you are vegetarian, you will love this version. Otherwise, you can add ground turkey, grilled chicken breast or ground buffalo for a filling, quick meal.

1 **THIN** BOBOLI pizza crust
1 jar of pesto or use the pesto recipe in this book
1 package of shredded Mozzarella
¼ cup Parmesan cheese

CHOICE OF INGREDIENTS:

Roma tomatoes
Sun-dried tomatoes
Broccoli
Asparagus
Yellow squash
Red or green onions
Chopped spinach
Red peppers
Garlic—chopped

PREHEAT OVEN TO 400 degrees

Spray a pizza pan with cooking spray and place pizza crust on top. Spread pesto evenly over crust. Add your favorite vegetables and sprinkle with mozzarella and Parmesan. BAKE at 400 degrees for 17 minutes. Enjoy!

125 calories per slice
3 grams fat
41 gram of good carbohydrates
4 grams of protein without chicken or turkey

Makes 6 large slices

SEAFOOD PIZZA

Any seafood lover will enjoy this quick and easy pizza. I like to keep cooked, frozen shrimp on hand or scallops work well too.

1 THIN Boboli Pizza Crust

Tomato-Basil Sauce from this book
2 cloves of garlic—minced
1 tsp. fresh grated lemon zest
3 tablespoons Parmesan cheese—grated
Cooked Shrimp—chopped into large chunks

Spray a pizza pan and place pizza crust on pan—spread with tomato basil sauce and top with shrimp, garlic, lemon zest and Parmesan cheese. BAKE at 400 degrees for 15 minutes. Enjoy!

225 calories per slice
5 grams fat
38 grams carbohydrates
12 grams protein

Makes 6 slices

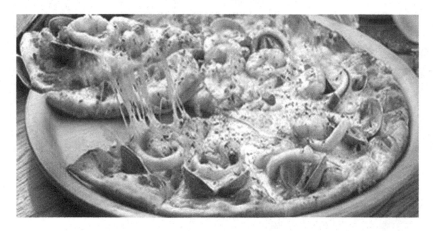

CARAMELIZED ONION PIZZA WITH BUFFALO

Caramelized onions and sautéed garlic add wonderful flavor to this hearty, but low-fat pizza. Serve with a side salad tossed in a vinaigrette salad dressing for a delicious meal.

1 THIN Boboli pizza crust
1 pound of ground buffalo
3 onions—sliced and separated into rings
6 cloves of garlic—minced
Pizza Sauce
3 tablespoons ground thyme
1 bay leaf—crushed
Sea salt and pepper to taste
Extra Virgin Olive oil
Mozzarella cheese—shredded
Parmesan cheese—grated

PREHEAT OVEN TO 400 degrees

In a large skillet, add 2 tablespoons of olive oil and cook onions until caramelized. Add garlic and cook through. Cook ground buffalo and season with sea salt and pepper. Spread pizza sauce over pizza crust and add buffalo, onions and garlic. Sprinkle with herbs, low-fat Mozzarella and Parmesan. BAKE at 400 degrees for 17 minutes.

185 calories per slice
4 grams fat
10 grams protein
26 grams carbohydrates

Makes 6 slices

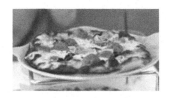

TURKEY PASTA BAKE

I always keep ground turkey, pasta made from rice and tomato-basil sauce on hand to make a quick meal any day of the week. You can combine all the ingredients and bake in the oven or combine the sauce with ground turkey and serve over pasta made from rice. Sprinkle with Parmesan

1 package ground turkey breast
Extra Virgin Olive oil
Sea salt and pepper to taste
Italian herbs
1 package of your favorite pasta made from rice
Tomato-Basil sauce from this book
8 ounces of Mozzarella cheese—shredded
Parmesan cheese

PREHEAT OVEN TO 350 DEGREES

In a medium skillet, add 2 tablespoons of olive oil and ground turkey—Season with sea salt, pepper and Italian herbs. Cook rice pasta according to package directions and drain. Rice pasta cooks in less time than regular pasta. Combine turkey and pasta and pour into baking pan coated with cooking spray. Sprinkle with mozzarella and parmesan. BAKE at 350 degrees for 40 minutes.

325 calories per serving
5 grams fat
31 grams carbohydrates
22 grams protein

Makes 8 servings

MAPLE MUSTARD CHICKEN

This dish has a wonderful, unique flavor and lends itself well to becoming a holiday specialty. The aroma alone as it bakes is fabulous! Instead of using maple syrup with the extra calories and sugar, substitute maple extract to achieve the unusual flavor. The extra sauce can be poured over pasta or a baked potato. Acorn squash baked in the oven complements this entrée well and you can serve the extra sauce on the side.

4 chicken breasts—boneless and skinless
Extra Virgin Olive oil
2 tablespoons Maple extract
1 large carton of low-sodium chicken broth
4 tablespoons Dijon mustard
1 tsp. ground thyme
Sea salt and pepper to taste

Coat chicken breasts in olive oil and season with sea salt and pepper. Heat a large skillet and cook chicken breasts about 5 minutes on each side—remove and keep warm. In same skillet, add chicken broth, maple extract, mustard and thyme. Stir and bring to a boil. Reduce heat and simmer 15-20 minutes—return chicken back to pan and heat through—serve sauce on the side or pour over each chicken breast.

195 calories
3 grams fat
24 grams protein
11 grams carbohydrates

Makes 4 servings

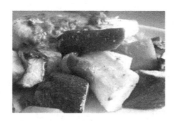

CRANBERRY CHICKEN

This recipe is another dish for a special holiday treat because of the cranberry sauce or you can serve it any time of year. Serve with wild rice and a vegetable and you are good to go!

4 chicken breasts—skinless and boneless
1 container of cranberry sauce
1 bottle of low-fat French dressing
1 packet of Onion Soup Mix

Combine sauce, dressing and soup mix and let chicken marinate in the mixture all day or night. Arrange chicken breasts in baking pan and bake at 400 degrees for 20 minutes or until done. Serve immediately!

285 calories
6 grams fat
22 grams protein
20 grams carbohydrates

Makes 4 servings

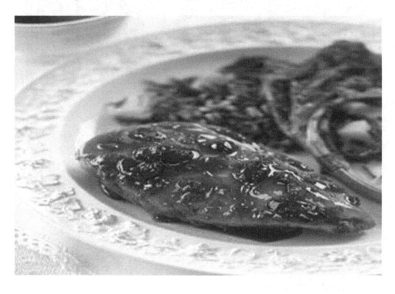

APRICOT-MUSTARD CHICKEN

This is an unusual combination of flavors that add some kick to every day chicken. Here is another way to eat low fat without sacrificing taste.

4 chicken breasts—boneless and skinless
1 jar apricot nectar
3 tablespoons Dijon Mustard
2 green onions—cut in a diagonal into strips

Pour nectar and mustard into large skillet—bring to a boil and add chicken breast. Cover and cook for 20-30 minutes on medium low heat. Serve over brown rice and add a vegetable or salad for a great meal.

195 calories
4 grams fat
24 grams protein
9 grams carbohydrates

Makes 4 servings

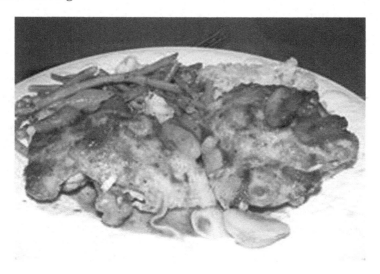

QUICK SAUTEED VEGETABLES

Your whole family will love vegetables sautéed in teriyaki sauce and vinegar. Experiment with any fresh vegetables.

1 zucchini—cut into chunks
1 yellow squash—cut into chunks
1 green onion—chopped
¼ cup red wine vinegar or you can use balsamic vinegar
2 tablespoons teriyaki sauce
2 tablespoons extra virgin olive oil
Pinch of sea salt
Pepper to taste

Heat large skillet on medium heat.

Cut vegetables and place in bowl. Add vinegar, teriyaki sauce and olive oil and season with a pinch of sea salt and pepper—toss well. Pour mixture into hot skillet and cook until desired tenderness.

35 calories per 1 cup serving
1 gram of fat
8 grams carbohydrates
1 gram of protein

Makes 2 servings

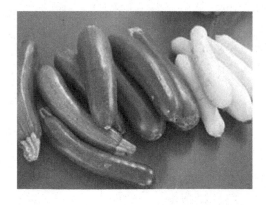

CHICKEN PIQUANT

This recipe makes one of those "party perfect" dishes that is easy to prepare and fool-proof every time. The sauce is best made in the morning and left in a blender until ready to prep the chicken.

6 chicken breasts—boneless and skinless
¾ cup Rose Wine
½ cup low-sodium soy sauce
½ cup low-sodium chicken broth
2 tablespoons water
1 clove garlic
1 tsp. ground ginger or you can use a small piece of fresh ginger
½ tsp. oregano
1 tablespoon of brown sugar

PREHEAT OVEN TO 350 degrees

Place the chicken in a baking pan coated with cooking spray. In a blender or food processor, add the remaining ingredients. BLEND WELL—pour over chicken, cover with foil and bake for 45 minutes at 350 degrees. Serve with wild rice and vegetables for a complete meal.

225 calories
6 grams fat
24 grams protein
11 grams carbohydrates

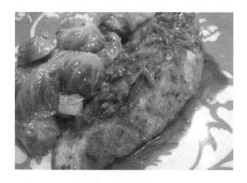

CHICKEN IN RASPBERRY SAUCE

Use fresh raspberries, when in season, or substitute organic, frozen, unsweetened raspberries to make this very different chicken recipe. A drop of raspberry liqueur will add extra flavor to the sauce.

4 chicken breasts—boneless and skinless
Sea salt
Fresh ground black pepper
Garlic powder
Extra Virgin olive oil

1 10-ounce package of frozen raspberries, thawed
¼ cup water
1 tablespoon of raw sugar
1 tsp. lemon zest
1 tsp. raspberry liqueur, optional
Cooking spray

Coat both sides of chicken breasts with sea salt, fresh ground pepper, garlic powder and olive oil. In large skillet on medium heat, add chicken and cook about 3-5 minutes on each side depending on how large they are. Remove and keep warm.

Press the raspberries through a strainer to get rid of the seeds. Place the juice in the skillet. Add water, sugar, lemon zest and liqueur. Bring to a boil, reduce heat and place chicken back into skillet. Coat with sauce and continue to cook for another 10 minutes at least.

210 calories
4 grams fat
11 grams carbohydrates
24 grams protein

Makes 4 servings

SPINACH-CHICKEN STUFFED BREAD

Stuffed breads make a tasty treat for a buffet table. Serve your family this fun and filling meal that comes complete with vegetables, protein and carbohydrates. No one will be able to resist the aroma while it is baking in the oven. This recipe is very quick and easy to prepare and makes for an easy meal on Halloween night.

1 package of bread dough
1 package frozen chopped spinach—cooked and drained
1 package cooked chicken breast
2 green onions
8 ounces low-fat Mozzarella cheese
2 tablespoons Parmesan
Pepper to taste
Cooking spray

Roll out bread dough on lightly floured surface. Sprinkle with spinach, chicken, green onions, mozzarella and Parmesan cheese. Roll up into a large oblong ball. Spray cookie sheet and place the dough ball on the cookie sheet—spray the dough lightly. BAKE at 375 for 30 minutes or until bread is golden brown!

Let stand for 5 minutes before slicing! Enjoy!

250 calories per slice
4 grams fat
11 grams carbohydrates
24 grams protein

Makes 6-8 servings

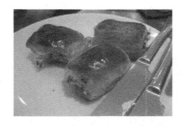

SHERRY PORK CHOPS WITH APPLES

Apples, dry Sherry, cinnamon and a little brown sugar add an unusual taste to these chops. Serve with Twice-Baked Potatoes (see recipe) and salad for a delicious meal.

6 Pork chops
Sea salt
Pepper to taste
Olive oil

3 large apples—sliced
½ cup Dry Sherry
1 tsp. cinnamon
¼ cup brown sugar
1 tablespoon of butter

Preheat skillet on medium heat—season chops with sea salt and pepper—add chops to pan and cook 2 minutes on each side. Remove from heat and set aside.

Slice apples evenly and place in baking pan coated with a little cooking spray. Sprinkle apples with cinnamon and brown sugar—dot with butter. Place chops on top of apples and pour dry Sherry over all. COVER TIGHTLY with TIN FOIL and BAKE 375 degrees for one hour.

250 calories per chop
5 grams fat
22 grams protein
11 grams carbohydrates

Serves 4-6

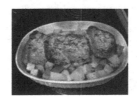

BUFFALO CHILI

Making chili with buffalo meat instead of regular ground beef cuts the fat and calories in half. Buffalo has 50% more protein and 40% less fat than ground beef and will fill you up very quickly. Ground turkey or chicken can be used to substitute for buffalo.

2 pounds ground buffalo
1 large can chopped tomatoes
2 green onions chopped or you can use a small yellow onion—chopped
2 tablespoons olive oil
1 16-ounce can of Baked Beans
1 16-ounce can of Kidney beans—optional
½ cup ketchup
1 tsp. chili powder
1 tsp. cayenne pepper
1 garlic clove—minced
1 handful of cilantro—chopped
1 tsp. ground thyme
1 tsp. ground dry mustard
Sea salt and pepper to taste

In large pot, cook onions in olive oil until transparent. Add buffalo and cook through. Add remaining ingredients and bring to a boil. Reduce heat and simmer for at least 20 minutes.

150 calories per serving
3 grams fat
28 grams protein
32 grams carbohydrates

Makes 10 servings

TURKEY BURRITOS

The Mexican favorite makes a filling, tasty and quick lunch or dinner. Use corn tortillas or whole-grain tortillas.

1 pound of ground turkey
1 tablespoon of olive oil
Sea salt and pepper to taste
Whole-grain tortillas
1 red pepper—chopped
1 red onion—chopped
2 Roma tomatoes—chopped
8 ounces of low-fat Sharp Cheddar—shredded
Picante sauce

PREHEAT OVEN TO 350 degrees

In a large skillet, add olive oil on medium heat. Cook turkey and season with sea salt and pepper. Add peppers, onions and chopped tomatoes. Place a tortilla on cookie sheet and spoon turkey mixture into tortillas lengthwise. Fold over edges and place fold side down in baking pan coated with a little cooking spray. REPEAT with remaining tortillas and turkey. Pour picante sauce over the top and sprinkle with shredded cheddar. BAKE at 350 degrees for approximately 10-15 minutes.

225 calories
5 grams fat
23 grams protein
12 grams carbohydrates

Makes 4 servings

CHICKEN FAJITAS

Again, whole-grain tortillas are best used for adding good fiber to this meal. Add some sliced avocado (about 1/3 per person) and low-fat sour cream for a delicious healthy meal.

4 boneless, skinless chicken breasts—cut into strips
Whole-grain tortillas
1 red onion—cut and separated into rings
1 red bell pepper—cut into strips
1 tsp. ground cumin
1 tsp. paprika
1 tsp. cayenne pepper
1 tsp. garlic powder
1 tsp. ground oregano
1 tsp. ground thyme
½ cup low sodium chicken broth
2 Roma Tomatoes—chopped
8 ounces of low-fat Sharp Cheddar
2 tablespoons olive oil

In a large skillet on medium heat, add olive oil and cook onions and red peppers. Add chicken breast strips and cook through. Add chicken broth and all spices and bring to a boil. Reduce heat and simmer until broth is absorbed. Serve with whole-grain tortillas.

225 calories
4 grams fat
11 grams carbohydrates
24 grams protein

Makes 4 servings

<u>CHICKEN QUESADILLAS</u>

Quesadillas is one of my favorite dishes to make—again use whole-grain tortillas and I keep PESTO on hand to make these any day of the week.

4 boneless, skinless chicken breasts—cooked and cut into strips
Whole-grain tortillas
Allow 2 tablespoons of pesto per tortilla
1 cup low-fat mozzarella shredded cheese
Sun-dried tomatoes—julienned
Roma tomatoes—sliced

Spread each tortilla with pesto then add sliced tomatoes, chicken, sun-dried tomatoes, and shredded mozzarella on ONE HALF of each tortilla. Fold over and press gently together. Heat a large skillet or you can use a Panini maker to cook each quesadillas. Use cooking spray to coat surface of skillet.

225 calories per quesadillas
4 grams fat
11 grams carbohydrates
24 grams protein

Serves 4

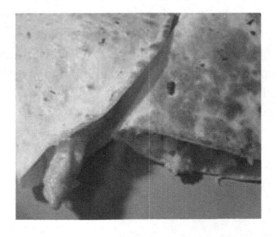

CHICKEN IN ACORN SQUASH

This is a tasty dish and makes a unique presentation for a healthy dinner party.

4 chicken breasts—cut into squares
2 tablespoons olive oil
2 acorn squash
1 red pepper—chopped
1 green onion—chopped
2 Roma tomatoes—chopped
Sea salt and pepper to taste

GINGER SAUCE:

2 tablespoons Dry Sherry
2 tablespoons low-sodium soy sauce
¾ cup low-sodium chicken broth
1 tablespoon of corn starch
1 tablespoon of brown sugar
1 tsp. ground ginger

Cut squash in half and place in a baking pan cut side down. Add about ½ inch of water inside pan. BAKE at 400 degrees for 45 minutes. Combine all the ingredients for the GINGER SAUCE and set aside. About 15 minutes before squash is done, heat a skillet with 2 tablespoons of olive oil—cook chicken. Add pepper, green onions, tomatoes and pepper to taste. Add ginger sauce and bring to a boil. Reduce heat and simmer for an additional 5 minutes. Spoon chicken mixture over squash halves and served with wild rice.

225 calories per serving
6 grams fat
30 grams carbohydrates
28 grams protein

Serves 4

LOW-FAT SHRIMP SCAMPI

The flavor of shrimp scampi without all the fat found in a traditional recipe can be enjoyed in this recipe by using low-fat substitutions. Serve with brown rice and vegetables for a delicious meal.

1 pound, uncooked de-veined shrimp
2 green onions—chopped
2 cloves garlic—chopped
½ cup dry white wine
Juice of one lemon
2 tablespoons olive oil
Sea salt and pepper to taste

In a large skillet, add olive oil and cook shrimp on medium heat until no longer pink. Add green onions, garlic, wine and lemon juice. Season with sea salt and pepper. Serve over wild rice.

120 calories per 3 ounces of shrimp
1 gram fat
11 grams carbohydrates
23 grams protein

Makes 4 servings

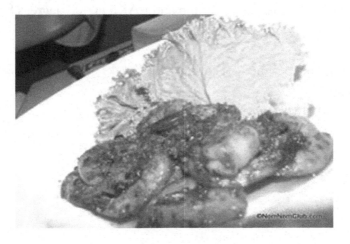

BAKED SHRIMP

Dijon mustard and a dash of red pepper sauce add great flavor to this baked shrimp dish without adding oil to the sauce. Serve with wild rice or whole-grain pasta and a side salad and dinner is ready!

2 pounds large shrimp—deveined and shelled
½ cup RICE bread crumbs—Italian
Cooking spray

Wine Sauce:

¼ cup dry white wine
Juice of fresh lemon
2 garlic cloves—crushed and chopped
2 tsp. dried basil or handful of fresh basil—chopped
1 tablespoon Worcestershire sauce
½ tsp. hot pepper sauce
2 tablespoons Dijon mustard

Coat a large baking dish with cooking spray. In a bowl, combine all ingredients for the Wine Sauce and reserve ¼ cup of the mixture. Set both aside. Add shrimp to the baking dish and pour the wine sauce over the shrimp. Combine the bread crumbs with the ¼ cup of wine sauce and mix well. Sprinkle over shrimp and BAKE at 400 degrees for 10-15 minutes until shrimp are cooked through and top is golden brown!

150 calories per 3 ounces of shrimp
1 gram fat
6 grams carbohydrates
23 grams protein

Makes 4 servings

SOLE FILETS WITH LEMON-YOGURT SAUCE

The lemon yogurt sauce adds a tangy flavor to the fish and helps keep it moist during cooking.

4 sole filets
½ cup low-fat yogurt—plain
Juice of one lemon
1 tablespoon Dijon mustard
1 tablespoon of horseradish
Cooking spray

Coat a baking pan with cooking spray and place sole filets on bottom of pan. In a small bowl, combine yogurt, lemon juice, mustard and horseradish. Spread mixture over filets. Cover and BAKE at 375 degrees for 15 minutes. Fish should flake easily with a fork.

95 calories per filet
2 grams fat
17 grams protein
5 grams carbohydrates

Makes 4 servings

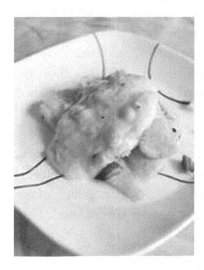

Chapter 13

Love Those Carbohyrates

Our bodies need carbohydrates for our brains to function properly. Carbohydrates provide the primary source of energy for all activity, both mental and physical. They are present in starches, sugars, fruits, vegetables and whole grains. Learning to control carbohydrates can be tricky and sometimes difficult to understand.

Unfortunately, the American diet has come to depend too heavily on the simple carbohydrates found white sugar, white rice and white flour. Foods made primarily with these are lacking in the B-complex group. Sugar is essential in the diet. The brain burns sugar for its fuel. A lack of sugar can directly affect the ability to think and function. A diet too high in simple sugar begins a roller coaster existence.

Think of the normal American breakfast of coffee, toast or worse yet, a sweet roll or doughnut or sweetened cereal with milk. A sudden flash of energy is felt, because the sugar contained in this type of meal is simple and requires little from the body to break it up and convert it to energy. However, with no nutritional benefits, a short time later, energy levels diminish as blood sugar levels drop. The metabolism is out of balance. Hunger strikes and fatigue is felt.

Sixty percent of each meal should contain complex carbohydrates that are rich in fiber, vitamins and minerals. An over-consumption of carbohydrates will cause the body to store any excess as fat for later use as energy. Weight loss can't begin until fat reserves are depleted. These recipes are designed for nutritional value and fat content and of course, taste.

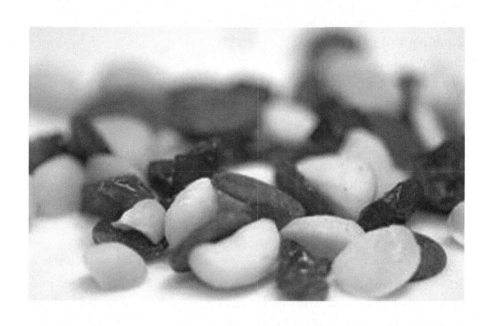

SPAGHETTI SQUASH PANCAKES

Spaghetti squash makes a colorful, low-fat side dish. The squash can be baked whole in a regular oven or cut in half and micro-waved. One squash yields five to seven cups of spaghetti squash for use in a variety of ways. Try something new for the family dinner! One pleasing way to serve this squash is for us in spicy, dinner pancakes. The flavor is unusual, low in fat, and tasty.

4 egg whites
3 cups cooked spaghetti squash
2 tablespoons ground ginger
2 green onions—chopped
Sea salt and pepper to taste
Olive oil or use cooking spray to cut the fat even more

PREHEAT OVEN TO 400 degrees

Pierce squash with fork and place in baking pan with a little water and bake at 400 degrees for 45 minutes or until tender. Remove and let cool a little before scraping out the insides strands of the squash with a fork.

In a large bowl, beat egg whites with wire whisk and add ginger and green onions—Season with sea salt and pepper. In a large skillet, heat 2 tablespoons of olive oil on medium heat. Spoon ¼ cup of the squash mixture for each pancake into skillet. Cook 3-4 minutes on each side. Remove and serve with low-sodium sauce for dipping.

47 calories per pancake
2 grams fat
12 grams carbohydrates
2 grams protein

Makes 4 servings

COLD RICE SALAD

This rice salad tastes best if refrigerated overnight before serving. Use a wild rice or any rice you may have or leftovers. This dish works well for a buffet because it is served at room temperature.

2 cups wild rice—cooked
1 pound mushrooms—sliced
4 green onions—chopped
3 tablespoons Red Wine Vinegar
1 tsp. Dijon mustard
Sea salt and pepper to taste

Toss rice, mushrooms and green onions together. Combine vinegar, mustard, sea salt and pepper. Pour over rice mixture and refrigerate overnight. Serve cold or at room temperature.

150 calories per cup
1 gram fat
44 grams carbohydrates
4 grams protein

Makes 4 servings

FLAVORED COUSCOUS

Couscous is Moroccan pasta found in most grocery stores in the rice section. Although a staple of the Mediterranean diet for centuries, couscous, only recently, has become popular with American cooks. It makes a nice change from rice, pasta or potatoes. Flavored with chicken broth, this ethnic dish is tasty and low in fat. Feel free to add green onions, mushrooms, peppers, red onions to the mix to jazz it up even more.

1 package Couscous
1 cup low-sodium chicken broth
Sea salt and pepper to taste
2 green onions—chopped

In a saucepan, cook couscous and green onions using chicken broth instead of just water. Bring to a boil and remove from heat. Cover and let stand for 5 minutes. Fluff with a fork and season with sea salt and pepper to taste.

45 calories per ½ cup
1 gram fat
32 grams carbohydrates
4 grams protein

Makes 4 servings

BROCCOLI BAKLAVA

Phyllo dough is fat-free, thin Greek dough found in the grocer's freezer. It is easy to work with because it comes in flat sheets and can be easily manipulated if kept moist. Spray the dough with cooking spray will also keep it from breaking up and will eliminate the need for a lot of butter. Other vegetables can be substituted for broccoli like spinach, for example.

2 tablespoons whole-grain rice flour
½ cup soy milk
2 tablespoons olive oil
2 green onions—chopped
1 8-ounce package shredded mozzarella
6 egg whites
2 packages of frozen chopped broccoli
1 package phyllo dough
Cooking spray

PREHEAT OVEN TO 350 DEGREES

Coat a baking dish with cooking spray. Stir flour and soy milk together until flour dissolves. In a large skillet, add olive oil and cook onions until transparent. Add flour mixture and cook until thickened. Add cheese and broccoli. Remove from heat and stir in egg whites.

Spray phyllo dough with cooking spray. In a manner similar to making lasagna, layer 2 phyllo dough sheets and then spread broccoli mixture gently over top of each pair of phyllo dough. End with dough on top. Spray with cooking spray and BAKE at 350 degrees for 35-40 minutes. Let stand for a few minutes before cutting into squares.

117 calories per square
2 grams fat
18 grams carbohydrates
6 grams protein

Makes 8-10 servings

STUFFED ACORN SQUASH

Try offering acorn squash once a week for dinner at home as a nice change from potatoes, rice or pasta. I learned to enjoy squash as a child and love its flavor and texture.

4 acorn squash
6 sweet potatoes—washed and pierce with a fork
2 tablespoons honey
¼ cup orange juice
½ tsp. almond extract

PREHEAT OVEN TO 350 DEGREES

Cut acorn squash in half. Place cut side down in baking pan and fill with ½ inch of water. Bake at 350 degrees for 45 minutes. Remove and keep warm. While squash is cooking, bake sweet potatoes on cookie sheet coated with cooking spray. Remove and peel skins off sweet potatoes while they are hot. I put rubber gloves on to do this! Place potatoes in mixing bowl and add orange juice and almond extract. Spoon into squash halves and bake in the oven for 20 minutes.

250 calories
1 gram fat
41 grams carbohydrates
7 grams protein

Makes 8 servings

TWICE-BAKED POTATOES

These are so delicious and they can be made with less fat and calories.

6 large baking potatoes, washed, dried and pierced with a fork
1 medium size carton of low-fat yogurt—plain
1 8 ounce package of shredded low-fat Sharp cheddar
2 green onions—chopped
2 tsp. onion powder
1 tsp. Lawry's seasoned salt
Pepper to taste
Paprika

BAKE POTATOES AT 400 DEGREES FOR ONE HOUR.

Remove and cut in half. Spoon potato out of each shell and set shells aside on cookie sheet. Combine potatoes, yogurt, cheese, green onions and seasonings. Spoon potato mixture back into shells and sprinkle each with paprika. Bake in the oven for 15-20 minutes.

110 calories
2 grams fat
22 grams carbohydrates
2 grams protein

Makes 8 servings

LOW-FAT POTATO SALAD

You will love this low-fat version of potato salad and it is quick and easy to make for a picnic or family gathering.

3 large potatoes—washed and pierced with a knife
¾ cup low-fat Miracle Whip
2 celery stalks—chopped
2 green onions—chopped
3 ½ tablespoons mustard
Sea salt and pepper to taste

For faster preparation, you could microwave potatoes on high for 5 minutes or I like to bake the potatoes ahead of time and place in the fridge to get cold and firm first—this way all the ingredients are cold and you can serve immediately.

Peel skins off and cut potatoes into squares. Add remaining ingredients and stir well. Chill and serve.

95 calories per cup
2 grams fat
22 grams carbohydrates
2 grams protein

Makes 4 servings

LOW-FAT NOODLE KUGAL

Noodle Kugal is a traditional, Jewish holiday dish, which is usually rather fattening. This recipe version continues the tasty tradition without the extra fat and calories.

1 package of noodles made from rice
½ cup black raisins
½ cup yellow raisins
2 tablespoons ground cinnamon
1 tablespoon lemon zest
6 egg whites
2 tablespoons olive oil
Sea salt and pepper to taste
Cooking spray

Cook noodles according to package directions and drain. Pour noodles into a large mixing bowl and add raisins, cinnamon, lemon zest, egg whites and olive oil—Season with salt and pepper. Coat a baking pan with cooking spray and pour noodle mixture into pan. BAKE at 350 degrees for 45 minutes or until golden brown.

75 calories per serving
1 gram fat
11 grams carbohydrates
3 grams protein

Makes 8 servings

POTATO PANCAKES

Potato pancakes can be enjoyed for breakfast or dinner. This low-fat version uses egg whites and bread crumbs made from rice to keep the calorie count down.

4 potatoes—baked and peeled or use 1 bag of frozen shredded potatoes
¾ cup Italian bread crumbs made from rice
4 egg whites
1 cup soy milk—plain
½ yellow onion—chopped
1 tsp. Lawry's seasoned salt
Pepper to taste
2 tablespoons olive oil
1 tsp. onion powder

Place all ingredients in a blender or food processor and blend until almost smooth. Heat a skillet on medium heat and add olive oil. When hot, add about

¼ cup of batter for each potato pancake into skillet. Cook about 3-5 minutes on each side. Repeat until all the batter is used.
35 calories per pancake
1 gram fat
11 grams carbohydrates
2 grams protein

Makes 4 servings

SWEET POTATO PIE

This is a traditional southern side dish and is quick and easy to make.

3 sweet potatoes—baked and skins removed
4 egg whites
1 tsp. of ground cinnamon
1 tsp. ground nutmeg
½ cup low-fat yogurt—plain
Sea salt
Cooking spray

PREHEAT OVEN TO 350 DEGREES

Coat a pie plate with cooking spray. Whisk egg whites, spices and yogurt together—add sweet potatoes and stir well. Pour into pie plate and bake for one hour. Let stand for at least 5 minutes. Cut into wedges and serve!

110 calories
1 gram fat
27 grams carbohydrates
6 grams protein

Makes 4-6 servings

Chapter 14

Sweet Endings

You can enjoy dessert, however, not on a daily basis. If you have cravings for dessert after every meal or at lunch or dinner, than make sure you are getting enough protein at your meal and enough fibrous carbohydrates, in particular vegetables and whole grains.

There is a way to have dessert without a lot of calories, sugar, fat or guilt. Use cocoa powder instead of chocolate or use dark chocolate instead of milk chocolate for more antioxidants. Use egg whites instead of a whole egg in recipes. Use low-fat ingredients as opposed to fat-free because they contain less sugar.

You will find gluten-free mixes in the baking section of most grocery stores for making brownies, cookies and pie-crusts because so many people are allergic to gluten—a highly reactive food found in wheat flour and wheat products. Substitute rice flour in some of your favorite recipes and take traditional family recipes and substitute low-fat products for ingredients. It will cut the calories and fat content in half.

PUMPKIN CAKE
with LOW-FAT CREAM CHEESE FROSTING

This low-fat version pumpkin cake is fun to serve for Halloween or Thanksgiving and tastes great with or without the frosting.

8 egg whites
2 cups rice flour
2 tsp. baking soda
1 tsp. ground cloves
2 tsp. cinnamon
1 tsp. ground ginger
1 tsp. ground nutmeg
½ cup sugar
2 tablespoons honey
1 large can of packed pumpkin

PREHEAT OVEN TO 350 DEGREES

Sift flour and soda together—add spices. In another bowl, beat egg whites, sugar, honey and pumpkin with an electric mixer. Add flour mixture to pumpkin mixture and mix thoroughly. Pour into greased Bundt cake pan and bake for one hour. Remove from oven and let stand for 10 minutes before removing cake from pan—let cool completely before frosting.

FROSTING:

1 8-ounce package of low-fat cream cheese—room temperature
1 tablespoon of vanilla extract
¼ cup sugar
Mix all ingredients well and frost entire cake!
180 calories
3 grams fat
3 grams protein
23 grams carbohydrates

Makes 10 servings

GINGERBREAD WITH LEMON SAUCE

Gingerbread is an all-time favorite dessert both to taste and to smell cooking. The lemon sauce adds a tart topping without a lot of calories and fat. This recipe makes a wonderful healthy, home-made gift during the holidays to be enjoyed by all.

1 cup of whole-grain flour
1 tsp. baking soda
¼ cup sugar
2 tsp. pumpkin pie spice
2 egg whites
2 tablespoons molasses
½ cup hot water
Cooking spray

Combine flour, sugar and pumpkin pie spice in a mixing bowl. In another bowl, combine egg whites and molasses. Set aside. In a third bowl, combine water and baking soda. Add molasses mixture and water mixture to the flour mixture and stir well.

Pour batter into an 8-inch baking pan coated with cooking spray. Bake at 450 degrees for 20 minutes. Cool slightly.

Cut into squares and serve with lemon sauce.

LEMON SAUCE

3 tablespoons sugar
2 teaspoons corn starch
1 tsp. lemon zest
Juice of one lemon

Combine all ingredients in a saucepan and cook over medium heat until thickened. Serve immediately.

120 calories per serving
1 gram fat
25 grams carbohydrates
3 grams protein

FRESH FRUIT PIZZA

Fresh fruit pizza is a wonderful dessert to serve on a colorful platter. The crust is made with egg whites and covered with a low-fat cream cheese flavored with almond extract. If you don't have time to make a crust from scratch, use sugar cookie dough in the refrigerated section of your grocery store. Use fruits that will not discolor like peaches, mandarin oranges, kiwi fruit, strawberries, blueberries, raspberries or grapes.

Pizza Crust:

½ cup butter softened
1 cup of water
¼ cup sugar
2 egg whites
1 tsp. vanilla extract
2 cups rice flour
1 tsp. baking soda
1 tsp. cream of tartar
Cooking spray

PREHEAT OVEN TO 375 DEGREES

Use an electric mixer and cream butter with sugar and beat until fluffy. Add egg whites, vanilla extract and water—beat well. In another bowl, combine flour, baking soda and cream of tartar. Stir into creamed mixture. Shape into a ball, cover and refrigerate for one hour. Roll out dough to fit pizza pan and bake at 375 for 15-20 minutes. Remove and let cool.

If using store—bought sugar cookie dough—spread out on a pizza pan coated with a little cooking spray and bake approximately 15 minutes until golden brown. Remove from oven and let cool.

FROSTING:

1 8-ounce package of low-fat cream cheese
3 tablespoons sugar
1 ½ tsp. almond extract

FRESH FRUIT PIZZA CONTINUED . . . .

For Frosting, combine all ingredients and stir well. Spread all over COOLED pizza crust leaving about one inch from the edge of the crust.

TOP WITH YOUR CHOICE OF:

- Strawberries
- Raspberries
- Blueberries
- Peaches—canned
- Mandarin oranges
- Kiwi fruit

110 calories per slice
3 grams fat
2 grams protein
24 grams carbohydrates

Makes 10 servings

DARK CHOCOLATE CHIP CHEESECAKE

Yes—you can make a low-fat cheesecake. This recipe can be adapted using a number of different flavors found in typical cheesecakes like amaretto, lemon, orange, chocolate and more. In other words, this is a basic cheesecake recipe that works with a number of ingredients.

1 package of Oreo cookies—ground in a food processor

3 eggs
½ cup sugar
3 packages of low-fat cream cheese
½ cup chocolate mini-chips
1/3 cup of dark chocolate syrup
1 tsp. vanilla extract

TOPPING:

1 large carton of low-fat sour cream
1/3 cup of sugar
½ cup mini-chips
1 tsp. vanilla extract

Press cookie crumbs on the bottom of a spring form pan coated with cooking spray. Place in freezer. Use an electric mixer to beat eggs and sugar for 5 minutes. Add mini-chips, dark chocolate syrup and extract. Pour into spring form pan and BAKE at 375 for 40-45 minutes.

While cheesecake is baking, combine all ingredients for topping and set aside. When cheesecake is done—remove from oven and turn it up to 400 degrees. Carefully spoon topping on top of hot cheesecake. SPRINKLE with mini-chips and RETURN TO OVEN for 5 MINUTES ONLY!

Remove and let cool for one hour—refrigerate preferably over night.

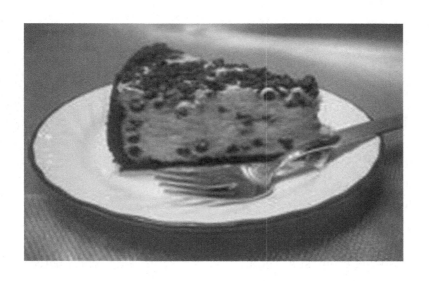

ORANGE CHIFFON CHEESECAKE

This is another great cheesecake recipe that is really very low in fat but full of flavor. Garnish with fresh orange slices for a special dessert.

1 cup of graham cracker crumbs
¼ cup canola oil
1 package of plain gelatin
¼ cup water
6 egg whites
½ cup of soy milk
1/3 cup of ricotta cheese
1/3 cup orange juice
2 tablespoons orange liqueur
1 container low-fat cool whip—vanilla

Coat a spring form pan with vegetable spray. Combine graham cracker crumbs with oil and press into the bottom of the pan. Place in freezer.

Dissolve gelatin in ¼ cup water and set aside. In a medium saucepan, combine milk, ricotta cheese, orange juice, liqueur, sugar, and gelatin mixture. Stir well over medium heat for 20 minutes. Do not boil mixture. Remove from heat and chill until partially set. Fold in low-fat cool whip and pour over crust. Chill until set and you are ready to serve. Garnish each serving with orange slices.

120 calories per serving
4 grams fat

Makes 8 servings

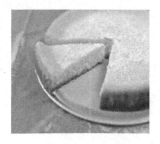

DARK CHOCOLATE
RASPBERRY FONDUE with FRESH FRUIT

This recipe calls for dark chocolate squares melted with raspberry liqueur. Serve with your favorite fruit for dipping.

1 large dark chocolate bar
2 tablespoons raspberry liqueur (Chambord)
1 tsp. corn starch
½ cup water
3 tablespoons honey—optional
1 tsp. vanilla extract
Pinch of sea salt

Place all ingredients in a saucepan and mix thoroughly over medium heat. Pour into a fondue pot and serve with your favorite fruit cut into chunks on skewers or you can use fondue forks!

20 calories per 3 tablespoons
1 gram fat

Recipe yields 1 cup

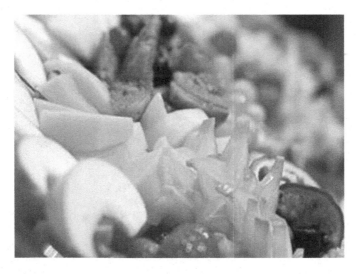

BAGS OF APPLES

This dessert tastes, smells and looks wonderful—it makes a fun presentation. It is like apple pie without the extra fat and calories found in the crust. Allow one apple per person.

1 package of phyllo dough
4 apples—cut into squares
Juice of one lemon
3 tablespoons brown sugar
2 tablespoons black raisins
2 tablespoons yellow raisins
1 tablespoon of arrowroot
2 tsp. ground cinnamon
1 tsp. ground nutmeg
1 tsp. ground cloves
Cooking spray

PREHEAT OVEN TO 350 DEGREES

Combine apples with lemon juice and stir well until apples are coated with lemon juice. In another bowl, combine sugar, raisins, arrowroot, and spices. Add to apples and mix well.

Place 3 thin sheets of phyllo dough on a cookie sheet and spray with cooking spray. Add 1 cup of apple mixture to the center of the dough. Gather dough up from all four corners and pinch together forming a bag! Spray with cooking spray.

Continue until all of the apple mixture is used.

BAKE at 350 degrees for 40 minutes.
195 calories
4 grams fat
38 grams carbohydrates
1 gram protein

To Your Good Health—

"Get In Shape FAST" is dedicated to helping you achieve ultimate health and vitality while still enjoying some of your favorite foods. Even though our program talks about getting in shape fast, remember to take it one-step and one day at a time. If you cheat during a meal, make a commitment to eat better at the next meal.

Find an exercise you will commit to doing on a daily basis. For variety, join a gym, take some classes, meet with a personal trainer or try yoga or Pilates for core strength and flexibility. Be good to yourself each and every day taking time out for YOU!

—Your Get In Shape FAST Team

For more information, visit http://www.getshapefast.com